Sociology and Nursing Practice Series

Margaret Miers
Gender Issues and Nursing Practice

Sam Porter
Social Theory and Nursing Practice

Geoff Wilkinson and Margaret Miers (eds)
Power and Nursing Practice

Series ISBN 0–333–69329–9

Series Standing Order
If you would like to receive future titles in this series as they are published, you can make use of our standing order facility. To place a standing order please contact your bookseller or, in case of difficulty, write to us at the address below with your name and address and the name of the series. Please state with which title you wish to begin your standing order. (If you live outside the UK, we may not have the rights for your area, in which case we will forward your order to the publisher concerned.)

Standing Order Service, Macmillan Distribution Ltd,
Houndmills, Basingstoke, Hampshire RG21 6XS, England

Gender Issues and Nursing Practice

Margaret Miers

First published 2000 by
MACMILLAN PRESS LTD
Houndmills, Basingstoke, Hampshire RG21 6XS
and London
Companies and representatives throughout the world

ISBN 0–333–69195–4

A catalogue record for this book is available
from the British Library.

This book is printed on paper suitable for recycling and made
from fully managed and sustained forest sources.

10 9 8 7 6 5 4 3 2 1
09 08 07 06 05 04 03 02 01 00

Editing and origination by
Aardvark Editorial, Mendham, Suffolk

Printed in Malaysia

In memory of my father,
William Edward Bluck
1912–1998

Contents

Series Editors' Preface   xi
Acknowledgements   xiii

Introduction   1
Writing and reading this book   2

PART I Understanding gender   5

1 **Approaches to understanding gender**   7
    Introduction   7
    Defining gender and differentiating sex and gender   9
    Gender and nursing   11
    Biologically determinist explanations for
      gender differences   12
    Key features of the concept of gender   13
    Explaining gender differences and inequalities 16
    The social functions of gender differences   17
    Marxism, capitalism and women's role in the
      bourgeois family   18
    Interactionism   19
    Taking gender seriously: feminisms   20
    Liberal feminism   21
    Radical feminism   21
    Marxist feminism, materialism and dual systems theory   22
    Black feminist approaches   24
    Postmodernism   25
    Taking gender seriously: studying men and masculinity   26
    Conclusion   26

2 **Masculinities and femininities**   28
    Introduction   28
    Masculine and feminine cultural 'codes'   29
    Identifying masculinities and femininities   31
    Woman as sex object   35
    Heterosexual masculinity: man as playboy,
      womaniser, stud   36
    Good woman   37

'Good guy', citizen, gentleman   38
'Bad guy': machismo masculinity   40
Explaining masculinities and femininities   41
Bourdieu and cultural capital   44
Nursing gender, ideological projects and cultural capital   46

3   **Gender and health**   **48**
Introduction   48
Mortality rates   48
Morbidity   50
Methodological difficulties involved in studying gender and
     health   51
Explaining gender differences in health   53
Women, work and health   54
Socioeconomic position and gender differences in health   55
Feminism, gender and health   57
Gender, cultural codes and health   58
Measuring masculinity   59
Masculinity and health   60
Masculinities, femininities and health   61

PART II **Gender and nursing**   **65**

4   **Choosing to nurse: from Florence Nightingale to
     the National Health Service**   **67**
Introduction   67
Nursing in the nineteenth century   69
Handy-women and private nurses   70
Nursing sisterhoods and Christian ladies   71
Female nurses in the Crimean War   74
Nursing hierarchies in nineteenth century England   75
Men in nursing in the nineteenth century   76
Male doctors and female nurses in the nineteenth century   78
Sociological approaches to nursing history:
     feminist accounts   79
Nursing and the labour market   79
Nursing in the twentieth century: 1900–45   81
Changes in health care   82
The effects of war: nurses, VADs and health visitors   84
The registration movement   85
Men in nursing 1900–45   88
Summary   90

5   Nursing in the NHS   92
    Introduction   92
    Women's changing role   92
    Nursing and women's changing work experiences   95
    Creating a feminine intellectual elite   98
    Class, curriculum and caring   100
    Nurses' relationships with doctors   102
    Men in nursing   102
    Men in management   104
    Masculinities and nursing   106

PART III Gender, autonomy and management   109

6   What do nurses do? Caring as a gendered concept   111
    Introduction   111
    Nursing care and the traditional image of the nurse   112
    Care and the intrinsic rewards of nursing   113
    Developing a caring self   114
    Gaining knowledge about care   117
    Gender, care and ethics   119
    Social science analyses of care   122
    Emotional labour, emotion work and feeling rules   124
    Summary   126

7   Dependence, autonomy and professional roles   128
    Introduction   128
    Gender and the development of individual identity   128
    Gender and emotional labour   131
    Caring, subservience and autonomy   133
    Emotional labour and the doctor–nurse relationship   133
    Autonomy and professional projects   136
    Challenging gendered cultural codes:
        a new professionalism   138
    Interdependence in health care   139

8   Gender and health care management   143
    Introduction   143
    The matron's declining role in the NHS   143
    Organisations and masculinity   148
    Men in nursing management   150
    'New wave' management   154
    Organising the organisation: gender and practice   157

PART IV Caring for men, caring for women   159

9   Gender-sensitive care   161
    Introduction   161
    Theoretical approaches   161
    Feminisms and gender-sensitive care   164
    Men's health and masculinities   172
    Masculinity and nursing   174
    Marginalised masculinities and health   176

10 Gender, identity and health   178
    Introduction   178
    Concepts of identity   179
    Adolescence, femininity and eating disorders 180
    Eating disorders and nursing care   182
    Gender dysphoria   184
    Masculinity and identity   185
    Masculinity and sports injury   185
    Masculinity and suicidal acts   187
    Motherhood and postnatal depression   189
    Professional strategies to support mothers   192
    Chronic illness and identity   194

11 Gender, power and sexuality   199
    Introduction   199
    Care of the body and sexuality   199
    Sexual identity and the experience of illness 204
    Disempowerment through health care   206
    Gender, violence and health care   209
    Sexual violence (and linked factors)   209
    Physical abuse (and linked factors)   212
    Men's violence to known women   214

12 Conclusion   217
    Gender, care and reciprocity   217
    Women as providers, negotiators and mediators
        of health care   218
    Men and informal care   220
    Caring in later life   223

References   226
Name Index   249
Subject Index   255

Series Editors' Preface

It is widely accepted that because sociology can provide nurses with valuable and pertinent insights, it should be a constituent part of nursing's knowledge base. To take but a few substantive examples, sociology can help nurses to understand the causes and distribution of ill health, the experience of illness, the dynamics of health care encounters and the limitations and possibilities of professional care. Equally importantly, sociology's emphasis on critical reflection can encourage nurses to be more questioning and self-aware, thus helping them to provide flexible, non-discriminatory, client-centred care.

Unfortunately, while the aspiration of integrating sociology into nursing knowledge is easy enough to state in theory, in practice their relationship has not been as productive as some might have hoped. Notwithstanding a number of works that have successfully applied sociological tools to nursing problems, there remains a gulf between the two disciplines, which has led some to question the utility of the relationship.

On the one hand, sociologists, while taking an interest in nursing's occupational position, have not paid great attention to the actual work that nurses do. This is partially the result of the limitations of sociological surveillance. Nurses work in confidential, private and intimate settings with their clients, and sociologists' access to such settings is necessarily restricted. Moreover, nurses find it difficult to talk about their work, except to other nurses. As a result, core issues pertaining to nursing have been less than thoroughly treated in the sociological literature. There is thus a disjunction between what nurses require from sociology and what sociologists can provide.

On the other hand, nurses are on equally uncertain ground when they attempt to use sociology themselves. Nurses are often reliant on carefully simplified introductory texts, which, because of their broad remit, are often unable to provide an in-depth understanding of sociological insights. Nor is it simply a matter of knowledge; there are tensions between the outlooks of nursing and of sociology. Because nursing work involves individual inter-actions, it is not surprising that when nurses turn to sociology, they turn to those elements that concentrate on microsocial inter-action. While this is useful in so far as it goes, it does not provide nurses with knowledge of the restraints and enablements imposed upon individual actions by social structures.

The aim of the *Sociology and Nursing Practice* series is to bridge these gaps between the disciplines. The authors of the series are nurses or teachers of nurses and therefore have an intimate under-standing of nursing work and an appreciation of the importance of individualised nursing care. Yet at the same time, they are committed to a sociological outlook that asserts the salience of wider social forces to the work of nurses. The texts apply socio-logical theories and concepts to practical aspects of nursing. They explore nursing care as part of the social world, showing how different approaches to understanding the relationship between the individual and society have implications for nursing practice. By concentrating on a specific aspect of sociology or nursing, each book is able to provide the reader with a deeper knowledge of those aspects of sociology most pertinent to their own area of work or study. We hope that the series will encourage nurses to analyse critically their practice and profession, and to develop their own contribution to health care.

Margaret Miers, Sam Porter and Geoff Wilkinson

Acknowledgements

This book has been written during a prolonged period of change and development in nurse education. I am grateful to colleagues at the University of the West of England, Bristol, for their support through the long hours demanded by the complexity of our work. They have, in many different ways, given me the confidence to write the book.

Richenda Milton-Thompson's support is a source of encouragement that helps to make writing a pleasure. I owe thanks to Sam Porter and Geoff Wilkinson for their time and commitment to this text, and to the series of which it is a part. Geoff Wilkinson's constructive reading of the chapters has significantly clarified many issues. I am grateful for the subtlety of his challenge and guidance.

Every effort has been made to trace all the copyright holders but if any have been inadvertently overlooked the publishers will be pleased to make the necessary arrangements at the first opportunity.

MARGARET MIERS
May 1999

Introduction

As the millennium approaches, nurses face challenges in changing services, practices and interprofessional relationships. Oakley (1993: 46) has suggested that for nurses to map their response to change, 'all they need to do is recover their past'. In recovering their past, they will recover their strength, a strength that lies in their alertness to the needs of others. It is a strength, as sociologists have often observed, associated with women. As such, it is denigrated as being of secondary importance to individual achievement and self-actualisation. Understanding both nursing's strength and its denigration involves understanding and analysing gender.

Sociology, in particular the sociology of health, illness and health care, has much to say about nursing and gender. Part I of this book introduces relevant sociological approaches to understanding gender, Chapter 3 examining the relationship between gender and health. Chapter 2 explores gender as a cultural construction through identifying diverse masculinities and femininities. Despite the diversity in gendered constructions of nurses as angels, sex objects and battle-axes, these images can be seen as collectively supporting powerful assumptions (ideological projects) about the (natural) social world. Heterosexuality, patriarchy and capitalism, for example, are linked together, sustained and supported through dominant, yet diverse, femininities and masculinities.

In recovering their past, nurses must recover histories that take account of the complexity of gender divisions and alliances. Part II explores these histories, including comparatively recent histories that have been strongly affected by changing educational and employment opportunities for women. Chapters 4 and 5 examine nursing's history not just as a history of women's subordination to men, but also as a history of the construction of different, often class-based, femininities. Gendered assumptions about the world are accommodated and reformulated differently by different social classes at different times, through an education system that has valorised the abstract and the universal, and through a labour market segmented by gendered assumptions about skills and careers. Sociologists are positioned differently from nurses in recent histories, an issue indirectly explored through reference to academic femininities in Chapter 5. Part III looks more closely at gender and care, dependency, autonomy and organisation. This section draws on Davies' (1995) important work developing a new model of professionalism, which would enable nurses to demonstrate and proclaim their other-orientation and their interdependence with other members of the multidisciplinary team. Lifting the veil (Oakley 1993) from care and teamwork, however, still leaves 'organising' in a shroud. Yet it is the continual and reflexive attention to detail in the monitoring of self and others that is the essence of nursing work.

Part IV uses varied sources of evidence to discuss the effect of gendered experiences on health and the ways in which nurses can use their understanding of gendered processes to enhance their care. Gendered processes affect self and other, constructing gendered identities, influencing illness experiences and behaviour. Gender is implicated in relationships of power and control, which can inhibit wellbeing (Chapter 11).

Throughout this book, I have drawn on a variety of sources. At the outset, I had hoped that a whole book on gender and nursing practice would allow exhaustive and systematic reviews of evidence about, for example, gender and health. However, recovering nursing's past, which seemed essential to any analysis of the present, took more space than anticipated. Hence the sources reviewed here, while eclectic and, it is hoped, indicative of the key issues, are not necessarily comprehensive. There are some major omissions, not least a consideration of gender and ethnicity. Another text in the *Sociology and Nursing Practice Series* will take ethnicity as its focus.

Writing and reading this book

Writing this book has become, for me, part of a reflexive project of the self (Giddens 1991). In recovering nursing's past, I have recovered my own. Giddens suggests that the trajectory of self has coherence through a cognitive awareness of the various phases of the life span. My social science-dominated cognitive awareness is tested by observations of gendered constructions of the social systems of which I have been a part. There have been many: education systems; families; health care; informal systems associated with interests, often children's interests. I have participated from different standpoints, depending on the stage in my life course – as student, researcher, teacher, mother, nurse and partner. In some roles, at different stages (mother, nurse, carer, part-time Open University tutor), I have been a mediator between systems and others' experience of them. In some roles I have been empowered by my position in the structure; in others I have felt oppressed. Such differences were related more to my structural position as part-time contract worker or full-time employee than to my skills or experience. My changing employment status derived from my family responsibilities. Three clearly gendered trajectories interlinked: my family roles and relationships, my education and my employment. Class position and early educational success are key factors in labour market survival, as are the support of partner and family. Gender is the key factor in career disruption and the costs of juggling family, work and study. Nevertheless, I have used continuing education to accumulate the cultural capital (Bourdieu 1986) most readily available to my gender and my class.

Hitherto, the troubling question in my reflexive project of the self has concerned the relationship between my own agency and the varied cultural constructions supporting social systems. The troubling answer has always been that it is only through participating in and moving between diverse social worlds that I came to understand the gendered assumptions embedded in each of them. I learnt through the juxtaposition of student and teacher roles, of carer and cared for, of oppressor and oppressed. It was friends' reactions when I decided to train as a nurse in my mid-thirties that made me recognise how deeply the academy denigrated nursing. Female colleagues asked 'Why?', 'Whatever for?' Male friends asked whether I would be wearing a uniform. An Open University student wrote in astonishment, 'Why should someone of proven academic ability want to become a carer?' The question still haunts me. Part of my reflexive project of the self, which includes this book, is to use my academic ability to seek to understand the mechanisms by which we sustain a culture in which that question can be asked. It is not just nursing's history that has to be reviewed; it is the history of all men's and women's professions and the history of higher education. It is the history of divisions *between women* and not just between men and women. It is the history of my education and my employment – the history of my ignorance – that led me, *as sociologist,* to ignore 'the importance of being a nurse' (Oakley 1993).

Yet I felt that I had always understood the importance of being a nurse, despite being so slow to consider nursing as an option for myself. Writing this book, exploring masculinities, autonomy, care and citizenship, I have come to understand more clearly some of the complexities involved in constructing my own gendered identity. When I gave the address at the funeral of my father, to whom this book is dedicated, I spoke of his sense of dignity and respect for self and others, of his infinite capacity to care; a gentle man and a gentleman. With such a father, I had failed to learn in my early years that caring was perceived as an attribute of femininity. I learned that later (even though I may not have been entirely convinced). His private care and public responsibility – fair and equitable in his treatment of family, friends, colleagues and strangers – may have shaped this book and my identity more profoundly than I can understand.

I would like to think that readers might use this book to reflect on their own femininities and masculinities, their own assumptions about autonomy, dependency, care and control, their own histories, and how they are shaped by our gendered culture, how structure inhibits agency. The cultural construction of both masculinities and femininities makes possible effective care within and across genders. That has been my experience. This book is an attempt to understand why and to encourage nurses to develop their own capacity to care in a gendered culture through enhancing their understanding of their own social construction as men and women, male and female, and as nurses. This book recognises the importance of nursing's response to, and participation in, social change. It is a tribute to the importance of being a nurse.

PART I

Understanding gender

1 Approaches to understanding gender

Introduction

The University of York student union alternative prospectus (YUSU 1997) tells potential nursing students that gender is an issue in nursing. Student nurses now take the presence of gender as a topic for study for granted and may be surprised to learn that, in sociology and in nursing, this was not always the case. In my experience of nurse training in the 1980s, student nurses were introduced to gender differences in mortality and morbidity without any critical reflection on ways of explaining or understanding these differences. Nursing's own gender imbalance was largely taken for granted. This chapter explores definitions of gender and key features of gender as a cultural concept before reviewing a range of sociological explanations for gender differences.

Sociology, like nursing, also largely ignored gender issues until the 1970s. Textbooks popular in the 1960s and 70s (Chinoy 1967, Worsley 1970, Broom and Selznick 1973) do not even list gender in the index. The 1975 British Sociological Association conference on sexual divisions and society was the first major acknowledgement by the discipline in Britain that gender had been neglected (Barker and Allen 1976). Abbott and Wallace (1990) argued that sociology's relative neglect of gender derived from the taken-for-granted assumptions of male sociologists who were interested in their own (male) experiences and accepted the gendered nature of social roles and opportunities without question. Sociology as an academic discipline was following rather than leading social change to address inequalities between men and women. 'Malestream' sociology had resulted in an emphasis on studying public spheres of social life such as government and the workplace, spheres in which men dominated; it tended to generalise from research findings based on all male populations and ignored issues of concern to women.

In the second edition of their textbook, which introduces sociology through feminist perspectives, Abbott and Wallace (1997) acknowledge that there has been considerable change as a consequence of feminist approaches. Feminisms' challenges to malestream sociology made a significant difference to many areas of sociology, including the sociology of health and illness, the sociology of professions and the sociology of work. Approaches to understanding sexuality, the body, identity and difference, among other topics, have been reconstructed by feminist sociology. The gendered nature of the social world is acknowledged and explored.

The defence of sociology's gender-blind (or malestream) position would be that sociology (like any academic discipline seeking to accrue knowledge in an objective, systematic way) was concerned with the identification of societal processes in order to explain the experiences of *all* individuals and groups in society, according to general principles and 'grand theories'. Thus, Marx's analysis of class could be applied historically and cross-culturally; Weber identified links between rationality and bureaucracy and between ideas and economic development, which could have significance across nations and epochs; Durkheim sought to define the nature of a 'social fact' and to delimit sociology as a discipline separate from psychology and biology; and Parsons identified the elements of social systems. As Porter (1998) makes clear, sociology developed through the logic of the Enlightenment, which saw the development of rationality as the mark of progress and civilisation. The liberal emphasis on the importance of individual rights as a means of maintaining individual autonomy supported a view that women's issues would be appropriately dealt with through extending the same principles of the rule of law that were supportive of the rights of man. A rational analysis of the logic of social systems was seen as capable of explaining the place of both men and women in a social structure. Sociology's rational analysis of nursing in the 1960s and 70s, therefore, emphasised nurses' relationships with doctors (Stein 1967) and the consequences of nursing's subordinate relationship to medicine for its claims for professional status (Etzioni 1969), without necessarily focusing on gender as a key explanatory variable.

Defining gender and differentiating sex and gender

One reason why gender does not feature in early sociology texts is because it was not until the early 1970s that gender was analysed as a concept distinct from sex. As Busfield identifies, gender as an analytical category was introduced as a challenge to biological determinism (Busfield 1996). A key text was Ann Oakley's *Sex, Gender and Society*, published in 1972. Oakley distinguished clearly between 'sex' as a term referring to biological differences between men and women, and 'gender' as a term referring to cultural differences. The separation of the concepts of sex and gender was important in order to make it clear that it is not possible to argue that gender differences derive automatically from differences in biological sex. Differences in men's and women's patterns of behaviour do not inevitably develop from the fact that it is women, rather than men, who experience pregnancy. The variation around the world and throughout history in men's and women's behaviour, and the variations in the degree of difference or similarity between men's and women's behaviour, wins the argument for a cultural definition of gender. Recent writers on gender take the distinction between sex and gender, and the understanding of gender as a cultural artefact, for granted. Books with 'gender' in the title do not necessarily include gender in the index (Davies 1995, Skeggs 1997).

Davies notes that her experience with student groups is that they have little difficulty identifying lists of sex stereotypes associated with 'man' and 'woman'. The lists of characteristics are culturally defined images of masculinity and femininity: 'Men are strong and women are weak; men are rational, women are emotional; men are active, women passive' (Davies 1995: 19). Early work on gender in psychology argued that the labelling of an individual as 'male' or 'female' occurs at birth, and an individuals' sense of being male or female follows through a process of socialisation into patterns of behaviour considered acceptable as aspects of masculinity and femininity. A sex-typing process was seen as leading to a sex-role identity. Research by Broverman and associates pointed to the existence of 'highly consensual norms and beliefs about the characteristics of men and women' (Broverman *et al.* 1970: 1). Cook (1985) has listed the characteristics stereotypically associated with each sex's traditional social role as:

Men (Masculinity) – aggressive, independent, unemotional, objective, dominant, competitive, logical/rational, adventurous, decisive, self-confident, ambitious, worldly, act as a leader, assertive, analytical, strong, sexual, knowledgeable, physical, successful, good in mathematics and science, and the reverse of the feminine characteristics listed below.

Women (Femininity) – emotional, sensitive, expressive, aware of others' feelings, tactful, gentle, security-oriented, quiet, nurturing, tender, co-operative, interested in pleasing others, interdependent, sympathetic, helpful, warm, interested in personal appearance and beauty in general, intuitive, focused on home and family, sensual, good in art and literature, and the reverse of the masculine characteristics above.

(Cook 1985: 4)

Cook identifies common threads linking the apparently diverse characteristics. One theme relates to distinctions seen as originating in family roles, that is, the distinction between male instrumentality and female expressiveness. The second theme relates to assumptions about the relationship of the individual and the social group. Masculinity is associated with agency, that is the self-orientated and assertive preservation of the individual. Femininity is associated with what Bakan (1966) called communion: integrated participation of an individual with the larger whole through selflessness, relationships and co-operation. Masculinity and femininity, in this sense therefore, are linked to fundamental questions about the relationship of the individual to the social group, the nature of consciousness and the nature of our knowledge of the world. Sociologists, in studying gender, have explored the links between social structure and individual identity, examining, *inter alia*, family structures, educational processes and the mechanisms of the labour market to understand how the social construction of gender differences reflect and reinforce established social structures.

Davies sees masculinity and femininity as 'cultural codes or representations of gender' and argues that 'gender, in this cultural sense, pervades our earliest experiences and shapes our sense of identity. Gender... shapes the way in which we relate to each other and structures social institutions' (Davies 1995: 21).

In this view of gender, masculinity and femininity as cultural products are clearly separated from individual men and women, despite the fact that it is through recognising stereotypes associated with the two sexes that our understanding of gender develops. In sociology, therefore, masculinity and femininity as cultural projects can be studied independently from empirical investigations involving the characteristics and behaviour of men and women. While there can be advantages in this approach, there are also limitations, particularly for attempts to understand gender issues and nursing. A study of gender that becomes disembodied and loses the connection with sex and sexuality would not be particularly helpful to health care practitioners.

Gender and nursing

Before moving on to explore approaches to understanding gender, it is worth reminding ourselves why gender is still an issue for, and in, nursing. York students' declaration that gender is an issue for nursing notes:

> there are more men in the profession than ever before, as more women are doctors... Students... live as other students might, although we have to work 37 hours a week, 45 weeks a year, which limits drinking time... Fitting in being an 'Angel' and those permissive sex orgies makes for a pretty busy diary...
>
> (YUSU 1997)

Gender is an issue because 90 per cent of nurses are women (Buchan *et al.* 1998). As a profession, nursing has been subordinate to the medical profession, which remains dominated by men. Nurses are both sex objects and 'angels'. 'Sexy nurse' images of nurses remain widespread in British culture. When teaching, I draw students' attention to a 'get well' card produced by 'Emotional Rescue' that declares 'I hear you're under the nurse' on the front of the card and 'hope you're back on top' inside. Many students argue this is 'only a joke' and harmless. Nevertheless, drafting letters of complaint, informed by different sociological approaches to understanding gender, is an exercise that challenges complacency about the gender issues nurses face. Men and women who are nurses live with the subtleties and complexities of cultural assumptions about gender, about nursing and about nurses' work on a daily basis. Denigrating stereotypes mingle with respectful and exemplary expectations, to be negotiated by individual men and women in varied work and social settings. Any reader, nurse or non-nurse, will already have some understanding of how gender issues may affect health and health care. There will be few readers who are nurses who have not noticed links between assumptions made about their profession, their gender and their sexuality. This book explores these links.

Biologically determinist explanations for gender differences

The widespread acceptance of the view that masculinity and femininity are cultural products does not mean that biological determinist explanations for behavioural differences between men and women can be entirely ignored. Biological determinist explanations have had a considerable influence on common-sense thinking. They derive from assumptions about the consequences of men's and women's differing reproductive functions. Physiological and hormonal differences between men and women and the different roles in child bearing are seen as leading to differences in psychological characteristics and to different social roles. Biological determinist arguments have been, and are, used to support the subjugation of women to men's authority. Arguments about biological inevitability can implicitly support men's superior status, if only through failing to question the social *status quo* as represented by men and women's division of labour. Biological determinist arguments, however, have been used to explain the differences between men's and women's social roles while still deploring the devaluing of feminine characteristics and women's work. For example, Mia Kellmer Pringle linked physical and physiological differences to temperamental differences, seeing women's nurturing capacity as deriving from their childbearing role. Pringle acknowledged that the positive valuation of masculine characteristics is culturally constructed, but she saw biology as having a part to play in the temperamental attributes of men and women, noting that:

> it may well be that because only women can conceive and bear children, they have developed a greater capacity for nurturing and caring which has then been further enhanced by the traditional division of labour between the sexes.
>
> (Pringle 1980: 5)

This may be a plausible argument, and an argument that may underlie some of the assumptions about gender and nursing already briefly illustrated. It may even be an argument that female nurses may wish to acknowledge and support since it brings coherence to undervalued roles, as mother and nurse, and suggests that women can claim an inevitably superior capacity to care. Pringle, however, offers no evidence for her assumption that temperamental differences follow from physical and physiological differences between men and women. On the contrary, her suggestion that male/female divisions of labour enhance certain temperamental characteristics is a suggestion acknowledging the importance of cultural codes and conditioning, irrespective of any possible biological imperatives. It is male nurses who are faced with a dilemma when confronting arguments about gender differences that link biology, nurturing, temperament and social roles. By Pringle's logic, male physical characteristics, their roles as father and in employment, lead to a temperamental emphasis on self-assertion, competitiveness and aggression, and an ambitious search for status. Although male nurses' career success may derive from assumptions about masculinity and hence become a gender issue in nursing, both male and female nurses (and their clients) also have to confront the gendered stereotypes that deny men a 'natural' capacity to care. It could be argued that a failure to acknowledge and notice men's as well as women's care, compassion, tolerance and reflective sensitivity denigrates men, denigrates nursing and impoverishes our culture. Equally, a failure to notice women's and nurses' ambition limits development for individuals and for the nursing profession.

Key features of the concept of gender

Busfield (1996) suggests that the concept of gender has five key features. First, gender is a *social construct* in that gender differences are constructed differently in different cultures and epochs, varying according to class, ethnicity and age.

Second, gender is a *binary category*, linked to the binary categorisation of male and female. The disadvantage of emphasising the binary nature of gender categorisation is, however, that it limits the recognition and acknowledgement of the diversity among men and among women, and the similarity between the genders.

The advantage of the recognition of the binary nature of gender categorisation is that it clarifies the importance of the *relational aspects of gender*. Davies (1992, 1995) is a strong advocate of moving away from the attributional approach to gender, that is, the listing of various dichotomous gendered characteristics as in sex-role identity literature. She advocates recognition of the importance of a relational approach, arguing we must 'talk instead about gender relations, as enacted through daily organisational practice and as about power' (1992: 230). The third key feature of gender, therefore, is that it is *relational*. Stereotypical assumptions about male and female attributes are made through processes of comparison, inclusion and exclusion. Men are stronger than women; women must be weaker than men. Women are co-operative and sensitive, but they are not analytical or strategic. The significance of a relational as opposed to an attributional approach is the acknowledgement that it is men and women who attribute gendered characteristics to each other. Men may notice and emphasise female nurses' sexuality and their caring nature; women may identify men's control but not their sympathy and support.

Davies's stress on the power dimension in gender relations reminds us of the importance of Busfield's fourth key characteristic, which is that 'the concept of gender typically, although not universally, connotes structural *relations of inequality, including inequalities of power'* (emphasis added) (Busfield 1996: 35). It is the continued recognition of the asymmetric power relation between men and women, men's dominance being contrasted with women's oppression, that ensures a continuing feminist concern with women's subordination. Nevertheless, asymmetric power relations can be studied from both sides, and there is a growing emphasis on a broader study of gender, including the study of men and masculinity. The emphasis on *gender* as opposed to *women* can, however, be seen as depoliticising the feminist project by broadening the focus and thus limiting or inhibiting concern with women. This book attempts to take a broad focus, exploring masculinities as well as femininities without ignoring the power issues that derive from the embedded nature of gendered assumptions in social life.

The fifth feature Busfield identifies is that gender is, using Connell's term, a *'linking'* concept (Connell 1987). Thus, gender stereotypes are not, as Davies notes, an 'unwanted import'

(1992: 230) that disrupts the egalitarian rationality of social life. Gender relations permeate social life and can be studied as integral aspects of social structures and activities. Gender is being identified as integral to an understanding of organisations (Pringle 1989, Savage and Witz 1992, Adkins 1995) and health and health care (Davies 1995, Busfield 1996). Gender is now not only a noun, but also a verb. Organisations, social relations and social practices are gendered, and the processes of gendering are being explored.

Despite, or perhaps deriving from, the extension and elaboration of the concept of gender, the initial distinction between sex and gender has been disputed (Edwards 1989). Criticisms of the distinction include the view that a clear biological male/female difference cannot be sustained in reality and that biological difference is itself a cultural construction that can inhibit the recognition of considerable diversity in male/female forms and sexualities. It can also be argued that the distinction between gender and sex supports an unhelpful Cartesian mind/body split, denigrating the importance of the body. As Busfield notes, these criticisms have been addressed by Plumwood (1989) through her recognition that gender necessarily incorporates a story of how the body is, and is conceived to be. It is the body that is the site of sexual and gender signification. Busfield (1996) is clear that the sex/gender distinction, identifying the cultural nature of gender, remains useful. My own view is that a sixth feature of the concept of gender could be that, despite the inherently cultural nature of gender, gender can be seen as being *embodied*. The gendering of institutions (bureaucracies, health care and education) can be understood through, and accompanied by, an analysis of the gendering of embodiment and the embodiment of gender, that is, how embodied men and women behave. It remains to be seen whether women as managers and men in clerical roles change workplace cultures.

An additional (seventh?) feature of current analysis of gender is the notion of *gender identity* (see Chapter 10). The recognition that the cultural construction of gender is linked to an individual's construction of identity has a long tradition in social science research, but psychological studies of sex-role identity (Broverman *et al.* 1970) initially dominated the literature and have been criticised for an overdependence on physiological differences between men and women. Early feminist explanations of gender inequalities in the 1970s have also been criticised for failing to explain the diverse experiences of women (Collins 1990, Bhavnani and Phoenix 1994). It is now recognised that neither gender nor identity is a concept that is easy to define; both are malleable and framed through diverse discourses, but constructions of gender nevertheless influence individual biographies through individual understandings of their self-identity. Women's studies, and the growing literature on masculinities, now take for granted the importance of recognising the feelings and identities of men and women of colour, or lesbian, gay and bisexual people, and of class differences in gender (Hearn 1992, Connell 1995, Mac an Ghaill 1996, Robinson and Richardson 1997). Chapter 2 explores constructions of femininity and masculinity in greater depth.

Gender issues in nursing are inseparable from constructions of the body, of health care relationships, of power and of sexuality. Nursing can be seen as a linking concept that links gender, care and health. Individual men and women, involved in their own identity work, can find that becoming a nurse problematises their own gender identity and that gender stereotyping problematises their identity as a nurse. Nursing, and individual nurses, are inhibited by the gendered nature of health and health care. It is young female nurses who may perceive themselves to be viewed as sex objects by those they work with and care for, and it is through the subtleties of their demeanour and professional relationships that the cultural constructions of femininity, sexuality and nursing are changed or confirmed. Sociology's attempts to explain such cultural constructions are reviewed in the next part of this chapter.

Explaining gender differences and inequalities

Sociological theories have explored the origins and maintenance of gender differences in relation to the origin and nature of family and work roles. Explanations have inevitably involved the analysis of power structures (such as patriarchy and capitalism) as well as analyses of the relationship between the individual and society and the constraints that culture and social structure place upon individual agency and experience.

The social functions of gender differences

The theoretical approaches that dominated sociology's development in the 1950s and 60s accepted differences in sex and gender roles as unproblematic aspects of functioning social systems. Parsons' (1951) concept of social role – a set of expectations and obligations associated with a social status or position within the social system – was central to his structural functionalism. In this approach, the difference in gender expectations, within both the private and public spheres, derived from the expectations and obligations of 'mother' and 'father' as distinct social roles. Since the roles of mother and father were performed by women and by men respectively, the attributes necessary to perform the designated roles successfully were seen as attributes of the two genders. As Porter (1998) explains:

> Parsons argued that values underlying any action within a role could be seen as either instrumental or expressive. Instrumental actions are those which are goal oriented; in other words, they are actions that are means to an identified end. Conversely, expressive actions are those which are performed for their own sake: they are an end in themselves.
>
> (Porter 1998: 24)

Parsons saw family values as being associated with expressive patterns of behaviour. Families emphasise responsibilities that derive from ascription, that is, from kin relationships and statuses (mother, grandmother) that are 'given' rather than chosen or achieved. Family members give priority to particular individuals within the family network (particularism) and are expected to do so. Such preferential treatment would be unacceptable in the public world of work and government. Work values of self-orientation, achievement and affective neutrality, however, could damage the stability of the family relationships, especially if individual family members came to be in competition with each other. Family responsibilities are necessarily collective and diffuse; parents cook, clean and clothe all their children. They cannot limit their responsibilities to specific functions as in the world of paid work. However, within the family, men and women performed different roles. Parsons saw women's function within the family as an expressive one, whereas men were seen as playing an instrumental role, providing the family with its means of support and decisive leadership. The domestic division of labour served both to maintain the stability of the family and at the same time to sustain the importance and the values of the world of work. Separating the public and private sphere, through maintaining gender segregation in roles, reduced the possibilities for conflict between expressive and instrumental 'pattern variables' (Parsons 1951) and the likelihood of conflict between individual men and women. Parsons' analysis of men and women's family roles links closely to the characteristics of men (masculinity) and women (femininity) already identified (Parsons and Bales 1953).

Davies has linked arguments about the effect of the dominance of the cultural code of masculinity in the public world to the professional dominance of medical men. Davies (1995) concludes that professionalism itself is a gendered concept and that the gender is masculine. She argues that nursing may need to seek its own professional development through deconstructing masculine models of professionalism and recreating professionalism along gender-neutral lines. Other writers have explicitly drawn an analogy between men's and women's family roles and the roles of doctor and nurse. Gamarnikow (1978) suggested that the doctor–nurse relationship paralleled the relationship between a Victorian husband and wife. Women, as wives and as nurses, provide expressivity under male instruction. These issues are explored more fully in Chapter 2 and Part II.

Parsons' functionalist approach to gender has been criticised for its 'malestream' assumptions, assumptions that saw a gendered division of labour between the public sphere and the private sphere as natural in the sense that there was a biological explanation for the link between women's role as mother and expressivity. The social organisation that preserved this link was seen as functional. As a result, neither biological explanation nor social structures were subjected to critical review.

Marxism, capitalism and women's role in the bourgeois family

Marxism became a major challenge to structural functionalism in the 1960s and 70s. However, the challenge was to the implicit emphasis on stability and social consensus rather than to the traditional assumptions about men's and women's roles. From a Marxist standpoint, the instrumental values of the male public world were bourgeois values that sustained capitalism as an economic system. Women were largely excluded from Marx's analysis because Marxism focused on wage labour and women were largely excluded from the paid workforce. Women's work was in the home, caring for the male workers and rearing the next generation of labour for the capitalist system of production.

Engels' (1985 [1884]) analysis of the origins of the family and the development of capitalism provided the basis for an analysis of women's oppression under capitalism. Engels argued that the bourgeois nuclear family had developed through the need to maintain economic power via an accumulation of capital. This led to the male need to ensure that property could be passed on to legitimate heirs. Thus, control over bourgeois wives within the home served the needs of capitalism. Zaretsky (1976) saw the changes in the place of production, moving commodity produc- tion away from the domestic setting to factories, as a main force in the capitalist oppression of women. Engels thought that the emancipation of women depended on their presence in the public workforce and on collective responses to the demands of childcare. These ideas informed Marxist feminist analyses in the 1970s and 80s.

Interactionism

Interactionism became a major challenge to structural function- alism throughout the 1960s. While retaining the concept of social role, interactionism stressed the dynamic social construction of social roles through role taking, negotiation and role making. Expectations and obligations can change through the unantici- pated consequences of action and reaction as well as through the conscious control and manipulation of symbols, most vividly portrayed through Goffman's work on interaction rituals and the presentation of self (Goffman 1969). Nevertheless, in identifying possibilities for individual creativity and control, and in emphasising the importance of a micro level of analysis of society, interactionists gave little explicit attention to women and failed to explore the significance of gender within interaction. This is, perhaps, surprising, since role taking and role making were seen as key factors in socialisation, and women's role in socialisation and expressivity had been noted and accepted among sociologists. 'Taking the role of the other' has been identified by social psychologists writing from a symbolic interactionist position (Stryker 1962) as being linked to empathy, insight and social sensitivity, attributes that have been linked to notions of femininity.

Interactionism, through the work of Mead (1934) and Goffman, illuminated the processes whereby interaction was linked to identity. Goffman's work on stigma distinguished between what he calls a 'virtual' and an 'actual' identity (Goffman 1968). 'Virtual' identities are ascribed by others on the basis of perceived characteristics, some of which, in some contexts, can become stigmatising and limiting in that they constrain possibilities for action and for meaning. In some circumstances, it is a stigma to be a woman or a man. Oakley's respondents in her study of housework were well aware of the constraining assumptions made about women who work at home and the consequent effects on their self-identity.

> I think of myself as a housewife, but I don't think of myself as a cabbage. A lot of people think that they're housewives and they're cabbages; I don't like to think I'm only a housewife... I usually say I'm a wife and mother and I've got a part-time job. People look down on housewives these days.
>
> (Oakley 1974: 48)

Although interactionism did not concern itself with the power of symbols that denigrate women (and nursing), it laid down some theoretical foundations that allowed the power of symbols to be explored. Interactionism fostered a recognition of the significance of the absence of diverse images. However, its neglect of gender can be seen as part of its lack of attention to structural aspects of power.

Taking gender seriously: feminisms

In exploring gender, it is feminism that has sought to link the individual to the social system, action to structure, gender identity to gender inequality, theory to practice. Sociologists who have used feminism to develop theories that take account of women have combined feminist and sociological thought in a variety of ways that result in a plethora of differing, if not competing, explanations of women's oppression. As Stacey (1997) has noted, 'feminist theory is not an object that can be neatly packaged and consumed' (p. 76). My packaging has been influenced by a wish to introduce ideas that will be useful in exploring gender issues in nursing.

Liberal feminism

As Porter (1998) identifies, liberal feminism is grounded in liberal political thought, which emphasises equality in individual rights to 'exercise their reason without hindrance' (p. 182). Sociologists writing from this approach have identified ways in which men and women have been treated differently, noting the way in which socialisation and sex role expectations diminished women's opportunities within education, employment, government and the law. Liberal feminists advocated legislative change to prohibit discrimination against women. Women, as human beings, have the same rights as men and are capable of full rationality. Restrictions that inhibit women's freedoms and accomplishments deny women equal rights. Liberal feminists would seek to remove and prohibit such restrictions. Porter notes Wollstonecraft (1970 [1792]) and Friedan (1963) as important writers within this tradition.

Radical feminism

Radical feminists argue that the most important division in society is that of gender. Women's oppression is seen as deriving from the 'the division of society into two distinct biological classes for procreative reproduction' (Firestone 1979: 12). Women's capacity for motherhood and the dependency of children on mothers' milk makes women vulnerable to the 'natural' aggression of the male. Such aggression may be used to control women, as in rape. Women's subordination is seen as universal and is sustained through the pervasiveness of patriarchy. All relationships between men and women are seen as institutionalised power relationships reinforced through all spheres of life, including personal relationships and sexual practices. Radical feminists thus see all relationships as political. Abbott and Wallace (1997: 33) identify three major issues within radical and revolutionary feminism. These are:

1. the relationship between feminist politics and personal sexual conduct, a key question being whether women can continue to live with men, or whether separation is essential;
2. whether sex differences are biologically or socially constructed;
3. the political strategy that should be adopted – withdrawal or revolution.

Radical feminist arguments have included the argument that reproductive technologies could be adopted to free women from the biological basis of oppression, thus leading to liberation. Suggested political strategies include living separately from men and celebrating the essential qualities, creativity and personal knowledge of sisterhood. Although the celebration of women's difference has had a widespread influence on feminist approaches to research, the reductionist nature of the emphasis on biological differences is problematic for many feminists. The emphasis on universality also detracts from an exploration of diversity and difference.

Marxist feminism, materialism and dual systems theory

Firestone's (1979) work on 'sex class divisions', which informed her analysis of the fundamental importance of the 'dialectic of sex', that is, the conflict between two biologically opposed classes of men and women, drew on Marx's analysis of social classes as forces of production and class struggle as the motor of history. Although Marx's analysis of the inevitability of class conflict and the overthrow of the bourgeoisie promised a redistribution of power, feminists recognised that lack of attention to women's role in society meant that change for the paid workers did not necessarily mean liberation for women. Women were supporting both capitalism and individual men through their unpaid work in the home. Women's role as health workers, both paid and unpaid, can also be seen as supporting male workers and the capitalist system.

Barrett (1980) developed a Marxist feminist analysis that included an analysis of male power within the analysis of capitalism. Barrett saw patriarchy as being shaped by capitalism through the development of a familial ideology of a 'natural' nuclear family with a 'natural' division of labour between men and women. Although the ideology of women's natural role as carer and domestic labourer predated capitalism, it suited the needs of the bourgeoisie and hence became established within the dominant capitalist class. From thereon, the processes of power and influence sustained through the relationship between the substructure and the superstructure of the capitalist system allowed the bourgeois family/household system to gain dominance throughout all classes. Thus, the interests of capitalism led to the development of patriarchal domestic relationships that themselves separated the interests of men and of women, inhibiting the collective strength of the proletariat and further supporting the interests of capitalism. Marxist feminists identified links between capitalism and patriarchy while retaining the Marxist emphasis on the importance of economic forces.

The emphasis on the primacy of class oppression as opposed to oppression by men has led to further debate and development in feminist analysis. Delphy (1977) has argued that women, within marriage, form a class that is exploited by men. 'To supply unpaid labour within a framework of a universal and personal relationship (marriage) constructs primarily a relationship of slavery' (Delphy 1977: 15). The analysis of women, as a class, in opposition to men, as a class, is a materialist feminist analysis, locating relationships between the sexes as originating from political and economic (material), rather than biological, forces. For Wittig (1979), women become a 'sex-class' in which sex acts as a signifier, locating women as women. Materialist feminists, therefore, use the logic of a Marxist analysis to identify the primacy of gender as opposed to class as the root of oppression. The difficulties with this position are similar to those of radical feminism. The emphasis on universality detracts from the exploration and understanding of difference between women. Furthermore, the ending of women's oppression may be, in this analysis, inextricably linked to the ending of heterosexual relationships.

Other writers have used a 'dual systems' approach to explore the relationship between patriarchy and capitalism. A recognition that patriarchy exists independently of capitalism – as men exercise power over women in non-capitalist as well as capitalist societies – leads to a recognition that explanations of gender inequalities in capitalist societies depend on an analysis of how patriarchy and capitalism interact. As Abbott and Wallace (1997) make clear, from the standpoint of dual systems analysis, 'to understand women's oppression fully it is necessary to examine the sexual division of labour in the domestic sphere as well as in the labour market, and the relationship between the two' (p. 41). Walby (1990) argues that, in capitalist society, patriarchy is exhibited through domestic work, paid work, the state, male violence and sexuality. Women's domestic work serves the interests of men not only in domestic settings, but also in work settings through allowing men an advantage in the labour market because of women workers' dual responsibility to the domestic world of work and to the state. Women's domestic labour has allowed men the freedom to develop new power bases in the economic sphere, leading to opportunities to create employment strategies that discriminate against women because of the structural disadvantages (in career terms) of part-time work and the segregation of women into lower-paid sectors of the labour market, particularly in labour-intensive and low-paid service occupations such as nursing. Assumptions about women's work extend beyond the domestic setting into paid employment, ensuring that highly paid instrumental roles within organisations remain within the control of men while women are relegated to roles demanding a more diffuse, expressive orientation. Patriarchy thus controls women in public as well as private spheres.

Black feminist approaches

Dual systems theory demonstrated ways in which gender inequalities could be linked with class inequalities to explore how patriarchy and capitalism worked together. However, black feminists have argued that issues of ethnic difference and of racism remain unacknowledged (Collins 1990). Black men and women have different relationships to the economic system from those of white men and women. Whereas white women and black women may share experiences of patriarchy, black women and black men share experiences of racism. Black men and women are sexualised and racialised in ways that make their experiences of being men and women in different cultures significantly different from those of white men and women. In Britain, the legacy of colonialism shapes the experiences of black men and women through, among other things, stereotypical assumptions about sexuality and skill. Racialised assumptions about gender and discrimination through employment practices have affected black men and women working in the health services, and racism affects the experiences of minority ethnic groups as service users.

Postmodernism

The search for the origin of gender inequalities explored so far are modernist projects that, in the name of progress, seek rational explanations for historical oppression. In contrast, postmodernism can be characterised by a disavowal of the possibility, or importance, of attempts to explain or analyse the reality of social processes or experience. Gender differences are not realities to be explored but discourses about gender that have been constructed. Discourses about gender can be deconstructed and the powerful effects of the discourses explored. Gender discourses are constructed through all cultural products: language, texts, narratives, representations, meanings and performances. In a postmodern world, men entering nursing change the cultural expectations of men and of nursing through their own performances.

Postmodernism privileges the recognition of difference in gendered experiences but problematises the analysis of women's oppression by denying the universality of women's experience as women. For many feminists, therefore, postmodernism must be rejected because it makes it impossible to use any binary category of male/female, woman/man without risking the accusation of essentialism (Busfield 1996). Nevertheless, postmodernist approaches to the analysis of gender and of sexuality may be seen as liberating avenues of analysis. Queer theory has analysed and celebrated the experience of homosexuality, identifying the centrality of homosexuality to the definition of heterosexuality and therefore of gender (Butler 1993). Recognising the diversity of sexuality releases the diversity of gender. Gender becomes performance, constructed and reconstructed through a multiplicity of meanings and sexual identifications that suggest a creative fluidity. In this performance, it is the body rather than a disembodied masculinity or femininity that is the site of the construction of meaning and identity. Postmodern approaches to gender issues help to celebrate the body within nursing (Lawler 1997).

Taking gender seriously: studying men and masculinity

Malestream sociology tended to accept male power as a natural, or at least a functional, phenomenon contributing to the stability of types of society, including Western capitalism. Whereas the dominant male analysis of patriarchy may be that it derives from a biological imperative, the analysis of men's gendered experience within academic literature has concentrated on the analysis of the complexity of patriarchy and of male domination, as well as on the diversity of experiences both across and within genders. Connell (1987) identified three structures that create what he termed a gender order: the division of labour, power relations between men and women, and sexuality. The links between the social construction of sexual relationships, the social construction of family relationships and the social construction of work relationships in paid employment are central to the analysis of the gender order. An important strand of analysis within masculinity literature has been the identification of what has been termed 'hegemonic masculinity', that is, an image of rational, independent, heterosexual, instrumental male leader, particularly dominant among the white, Western middle classes. Such a class-based image of masculinity oppressed men as well as women. The analysis of masculinities and femininities is the subject matter of Chapter 2.

Conclusion

An understanding of gender issues, including ways of understanding gender and explaining gender inequalities in society and in health is important to nursing because 'nurse' is a powerfully gendered symbol. A gendered culture attributes meaning to nursing through complex processes that are explored throughout this book. Surrounded by the powerful images of nursing and sexuality, readily available in the media and on greetings cards, nurses negotiate their own identities and act in the world as embodied professionals offering care and support to promote, maintain and restore health. Nurses care for vulnerable minds and bodies, minds and bodies that are weakened and strengthened by gendered processes. The processes by which nurses' work is devalued and denigrated are gendered processes, and the potential of gender as a linking concept in the analysis of health care has yet to be fully explored. Nurses, as providers of care and support, are central to an analysis of gender and health care.

2 Masculinities and femininities

Introduction

We have already identified stereotypes of women that are peculiarly linked to nursing. Nurses are sexy; nurses are angels. Recognising the importance of links between nursing and the cultural construction of femininity is not new (Garmarnikow 1978). Social science literature on the health professions has explored the embedded nature of gender within and between health care occupations (Witz 1992, Carpenter 1993; see Parts II and III). Davies and Rosser (1986) have examined the careers of men and women in nursing and the gendering of the concept of career. Nurses' work has been explored through an analysis of emotional labour (James 1989, Smith 1992), and care and caring have been considered in the context of gender and approaches to moral reasoning (Gilligan 1982; see also Chapter 6).

Davies' (1995) work has demonstrated ways of understanding the processes of embedding gendered assumptions in institutional and cultural life. She has suggested that there are masculine and feminine cultural 'codes' that sustain binary thinking about gender and affect social relations, affirming the value of characteristics seen as being associated with men. Women's activities and skills are thereby devalued and ignored; women remain marginal and misunderstood. Despite the existence of cultural codes, however, Davies acknowledges that gender is a 'social fiction' that is not sustainable as a basis for daily practice (Davies 1995: 185). Male and female nurses caring for male and female clients can both challenge and sustain this social fiction in their daily practice as a nurse.

Kuhse (1997), a nurse writing about nurses, women, ethics and caring, acknowledges the power of the social fiction, noting that 'the understanding of nursing as a natural extension of a woman's role means that there are close historical links between the status of women in a given society and the status of nurses and of nursing' (Kuhse 1997: 14). In nursing, understanding gender issues and women's role in social structures may be seen as a prerequisite for challenge and change.

The key features of gender already identified in Chapter 1 can help this understanding. Gender is *socially and culturally constructed,* but the difference between men and women may be more easily emphasised than the similarities because of the *binary* categorisation of male and female. It is the *relational* aspects of gender that reinforce the binary categories. Men's and women's different social roles lead to social relationships that may be structured around those roles, In the *social structure*, men have public, authoritative positions of control, but their dominance, activity, decisiveness and power depend on social actors, including women, accepting their authority and the consequences of their decisions. Relationships are *unequal*. Men manage, women are managed; men control, women obey. In the private sphere of domestic labour and personal relationships, however, women develop skills in the intimacy of care and support, which become the cultural property of women as opposed to men. The salience of gender constructions for individuals and their *identities* may mean that challenges to gendered cultural codes can be seen as challenges to personal identity. It is not in the interests of individual (*embodied*) men who value their own managerial and decision making skills to take notice of the co-operative problem solving approach of (*embodied*) women subordinates. If skills and actions are not equally valued, for whatever reason, associating men and women with different skills and actions can reinforce inequalities.

Masculine and feminine cultural 'codes'

Davies (1995) attempts to challenge cultural constructions of gender by using positive terms to present the cultural codes of femininity as well as masculinity. In re-presenting Davies' cultural codes of gender here, I acknowledge the danger in further reinforcing gender archetypes and stereotypes, thus sustaining the social fiction, but, like Davies, I would argue that in order to examine gender representations and attempt to understand their consequences for health and for nursing, these representations have to be invoked.

Davies has identified cultural codes of gender associated with the development of the self (explored in Chapter 7), with cognitive orientation and with relational style. The development of the masculine self is characterised by separation, boundedness, responsibility to self, self-esteem and self-love; the development of the feminine self by connectedness, responsibility to others, selflessness and self-sacrifice. The masculine code of cognitive orientation is associated with abstract, rule-governed thinking, mastery, control, expertise, skills and knowledge; feminine cognitive orientation is concrete and contextual, emphasising understanding, experience and skills and knowledge 'confirmed in use'. The masculine relational style is decisive, interrogative, agentic, instrumental, hierarchy orientated and loyal to superordinates; the feminine relational style is reflective, accommodative, facilitative, expressive, loyal to principles and group-orientated (Davies 1995: 27).

Cultural codes of gender, however, derive from cultural expectations about social roles, about the body and about sexuality. It is the way in which social structure, culture and ideologies shape social roles, sexual behaviour and relationships associated with reproduction and childrearing that lead to dominant (yet fictitious) femininities and masculinities. In hierarchical social structures that are shaped by capitalism and patriarchy, dominant codes of hegemonic masculinities and femininities, associated with dominant classes and the dominant white race, co-exist alongside diverse alternative constructions (black, working class, gay, lesbian) of masculinity or femininity. Hegemony is a term that derives from Gramsci's (1971) analysis of class relationships and refers to a form of power characterised by widespread consensus surrounding ideas that serve the interests of a particular group (or, as in patriarchy, a particular gender). Hegemony is achieved when a range of groups and interests accept ideas and practices as normal, even though such ideas and practices may, for some groups, contribute to their disempowerment.

Connell (1987) has adapted Gramsci's approach to analysing hegemony in capitalist society to the analysis of what he terms the 'gender order'. The gender order rests on the division of labour, on power relations between men and women and on sexuality. Cultural expectations of men and women deriving from, and shaping, men's and women's roles in reproduction and in the labour force sustain this gender order. Connell uses the term 'hegemonic masculinity' to analyse the process whereby ideological constructions of masculinity serve the interests of dominant male groups, perpetuating domination over women as well as control over less powerful men. There are however a range of dominant constructions of male and female behaviour – of masculinities and femininities – that constrain men and women in public and private settings. Aligning an analysis of power alongside the identification of a range of gender stereotypes leads to an exploration of the 'ideological projects' supported by constructions of masculinities and femininities. Different masculinities and femininities support different 'ideological projects'. Before exploring these 'ideological projects', however, it would be helpful to identify some masculinities and femininities that have particular significance for nursing and for health.

Identifying masculinities and femininities

Mother

Of all the images of womanhood available to women, none is more dominant than that of the mother. 'Mother', as a social role or constructed identity as opposed to a biological function, has been particularly clearly, and influentially, delineated during the nineteenth and twentieth centuries. Dally (1982) points out that 'motherhood' as a concept did not appear to exist until the Victorian era, when the idea and status of motherhood became linked to an idealised picture of womanhood as involving passivity and submissiveness. 'Motherhood' has been constructed by the changing needs of societies for men's and women's labour and by changing perceptions of the needs of children – but rarely by the needs of women. Whereas in Britain, state nurseries were set up during World War Two, enabling mothers to take on work roles while men served in the armed forces, after the war, as men returned to peacetime work roles, women were encouraged to return to the domestic setting. Bowlby's (1953) theories of maternal deprivation, emphasising the negative consequences of maternal separation for children, contributed to the pressure to return women to mothering in the domestic setting. Bowlby's views about the importance of the presence of the mother combined with views about the 'naturalness' of motherhood to confirm the centrality of motherhood for women. Richardson (1993) identifies the popularising of the ideas of Donald Winnicott through women's magazines and BBC broadcasts as being indicative of the view 'that a woman becomes an ordinary devoted mother just by being herself' (Richardson 1993: 45). Nevertheless, women are not always trusted to 'know' how to be a mother. Childrearing advice in the 1920s and 30s suggested that mothers needed expert advice about childcare, provided by childrearing manuals and by professionals, including health visitors.

The notion of ordinary, natural motherhood and the view that natural mothers knew that they must not be separated from their children has contributed significantly to the cultural code of femininity in Britain. It is women who are responsible for others – selfless, intuitive, caring. As Richardson notes:

> the experience of motherhood is highly complex. It is not just the experience of looking after and caring for a child. It is also an identity which, in our society is necessary for full status as a 'normal' and 'feminine' woman. To have children is to be a 'good girl' and is rewarded by social approval and social acceptance, providing of course that you are not a lesbian and unmarried.
>
> (Richardson 1993: 1)

Being a mother brings, for many women, a sense of belonging to the category 'woman'; motherhood brings a sense of maturity, a sense of purpose, of importance and of responsibility.

Motherhood as a social role, however, far from bringing the gains anticipated, has been shown to bring with it considerable domestic labour associated with childcare and, as Richardson argues, 'important social and psychological losses' (1993: 5). The losses were identified by Oakley (1979) as deriving from a loss of employment, of status, of independence, of privacy, of social networks, of personal identity and of individuality. Many of these 'losses' can be seen as the result of acting in accordance with traditional expectations concerning the role of the mother. Although the extent to which women now return to work after maternity leave indicates that a mother's constant presence is not now seen as being necessary, this does not diminish the societal emphasis on a mother's duty to care. The responsibilities of motherhood lead to the development of a caring self, produced through care for others. This selflessness can be seen as a gendered attribute, bringing strengths and weaknesses for women.

The idealised view of motherhood not only constrains our recognition of the negative aspects of the role, but also creates deviant mothers and can have negative consequences for health (see Chapter 10). Social science and feminist research have illuminated the ways in which single mothers, young mothers, lesbian mothers and black mothers have been controlled, labelled and ignored (Macintyre 1976, Collins 1990, Phoenix 1991, Romans 1992). Nicolson (1997) sees the central role of motherhood and her 'mythological, mysterious and powerful status' (p. 375) as a patriarchal myth ensuring that when women cannot perform the role to perfection, it is mothers who are blamed.

The patriarchal myth is also racist, negating the legitimacy of alternative models of motherhood. Collins (1990) has described ways in which black women share responsibility for childrearing, acting as 'other mothers' for each other's children. Understanding complexity and variation in the construction of motherhood is important for health care professionals, not just for their work with women, but also to understand the complexity of their own role as midwives, nurses or health visitors.

Housewife

A role often associated with the role of mother is that of housewife, a role that Oakley (1974) identified as bringing mental health costs. Feminist approaches, particularly Marxist feminism (see Chapter 1), however, note the economic value of women's domestic labour both to a capitalist and a patriarchal society. It may be the children's dependency on the mother and the economic dependency of women on men that lead to the paradoxical strength and subservience of motherhood when linked to the housewife role. Mothers are both dependent and depended upon.

Father

Whereas motherhood is closely linked to the social construction of 'woman', the social status of being a father has been less central in constructions of masculinity. Seidler (1988), however, has noted the associations in Western culture between 'visions of authority' and 'conceptions of the father' (p. 272). Judaism and Christianity ensure that authority is seen as being associated with God the Father, and seventeenth century Enlightenment ideas concerning reason and freedom added male political authority to the domain assumptions of a patriarchal society. Seidler draws upon Kant's arguments to explore the influence of assumptions about fatherhood that stem from Enlightenment philosophy:

> Within an Enlightenment tradition reason is set in fundamental opposition to nature – our emotions, feelings and desires. In the family the father is to be the source of reason. He is also to be the source of discipline.

> (Seidler 1988: 274)

The duties of fathering were seen as educating children to control their feelings and to accept behavioural control based on rational principles. 'So it is that fathers learn not to listen to what their children have to say, for this is not the voice of reason' (Seidler 1988: 297). It is fathers who have been presented as the voice of reason.

A new interest in fatherhood on the part of men can be seen as a challenge to these Enlightenment assumptions, assumptions that have also been challenged through male insecurity in the workforce and hence in the traditional provider role. The male (father) role in the family was traditionally seen as that of provider, head of the household. In a service economy, some of the particularities of masculinity, such as physical strength, no longer necessarily bring public roles in the world of work. If the provider role is challenged through a decline in the number of 'male' jobs and increased competition from women, a reconstructed role of 'father', allowing more involvement with children, may be more desirable as a part of a positive male self-identity. Canadian research concerning the effects of paid and unpaid work on nurses' wellbeing, however, has identified that, for male nurses, the parental role was important in diminishing negative wellbeing. The authors conclude that 'children contribute to the positive wellbeing of men and appear to diminish the chances of women experiencing negative wellbeing' (Walters *et al.* 1997: 340). Male nurses, however, could not be seen as conforming to hegemonic masculinity.

Woman as sex object

The smiling image of the nurse on the 'Emotional Rescue' get well card referred to in Chapter 1, the 'come on' smile of the page 3 girl, the face of Marilyn Monroe, are all familiar, and frequent, representations of women that are, as Winship (1983) makes clear, sexualised. This image of femininity signals availability, sexuality and glamour. This is what Spence *et al.* (1978) has described as 'the Look' created by the media – 'the full faced come-on, a full frontal attack' (p. 7). The sexy nurse is an image of women constructed through the male gaze. But women are also the 'consumers' of the image.

Media images of women, even when less overtly sexualised, often construct a femininity to attract men. Berger's argument is that in photographic imagery

> *men* act and *women* appear: Men look at women. Women watch themselves being looked at. This determines not only most relations between men and women but also the relation of women to themselves. The surveyor of women in herself is male: the surveyed female. Thus she turns herself into an object – and most particularly an object of vision: a sight.
>
> (Berger 1972: 47)

Thus, images of women constructed by and for men have become cultural codes of femininity and are hence images of women for women. Lees (1986, 1993) has explored how adolescent girls show their femininity by behaviour attractive to men and by dressing up. Skeggs (1997), however, has explored the ways in which girls use glamour as 'a performance of femininity *with* strength' (Skeggs 1997: 111). Glamour, for the working-class girls in Skeggs' study was 'a way of holding together sexuality and respectability' (p. 110) in a way that was difficult to achieve. For women, the contrast between sexuality and respectability is linked to a familiar contrast between Madonna and whore, between 'good girl' and 'fallen woman'. As is now widely recognised, gender expectations and attributes are framed 'within the context of compulsory heterosexuality… It is clear for example, that the meanings both of being a "good girl" and of being a "real boy" are constituted within a silent heterosexuality, which is made all the more powerful by its very silence' (Epstein 1996: 206). Smart (1996) has noted that woman as heterosexual *subject* is absent from feminist sociological literature. Heterosexual women do not write about their own sexuality. Within heterosexual relationships, women are perceived as passive objects of desire. As such, an analysis of gender and nursing may be similarly constrained by an absence of nurses' discussion of their own and clients' sexuality. There is, however, a growing literature within nursing on caring for gay men and lesbians (Godfrey 1999).

Heterosexual masculinity: man as playboy, womaniser, stud

If women are presented as sexual objects, it is men who are expected to desire them. Hence Don Juan and Casanova have been presented as models of successful men, successful in their sexual conquest of women. The language of supremacy and domination permeates descriptions of the cultural construction of masculinity.

Brannon (1976) characterised masculinity, or masculinities, as 'No Sissy Stuff', the 'Big Wheel', the 'Sturdy Oak' and 'Give 'em Hell'. Research on men's health (reviewed in Chapter 3 and Part IV) illustrates ways in which a 'Give 'em Hell' approach to life may incur health risks through behaviours such as hard drinking and fast driving. The 'Sturdy Oak' need to be independent and self-reliant can lead to delay in acknowledging symptoms of ill health. The physicality necessary to signify 'No Sissy Stuff' – a clear separation from the female form – leads to an emphasis on male strength and muscularity. Physical competitiveness through fighting and sport, therefore, becomes an important part of the construction of hegemonic masculinity.

Whereas feminist writers may concentrate on the way in which the male control of sporting images reinforces the subordination of women (Hargreaves 1994), gay scholarship has made clear the way in which the subordination of women is intricately linked to homophobia. 'Feminine' signs, used by men or by women, indicate a subservient position in the gender order. Hegemonic masculinity is heterosexual. It excludes and problematises homosexuality, for men and for women. Gay men and lesbians are constructed as deviant (Pronger 1990).

Good woman

An overemphasis on gender constructions as heterosexual ideology would, however, oversimplify their complexity. Whereas being a good father may not be an inevitable part of the positive construction of manhood, being a 'good mother' and a 'good woman' have been almost synonymous. 'Good woman', 'good mother' and 'good girl' are all constructs associated with respectability and responsibility, attributes associated with nurses as well as mothers. The good mother/nurse/woman analogy, however, attributed to Nightingale, is more complex than a simplistic view that nursing and motherhood come naturally to women. Nightingale's 'good woman' was a woman of high moral character. Nightingale's nurses were a 'higher class' of women, motivated by a dedication to the performance of good works. Nightingale's good woman/good nurse was in distinct contrast to those women carrying out nursing activities, stereotyped through Dickens' character Sarah Gamp, described by Nightingale as women who were 'too old, too weak, too drunken, too stolid, or too bad to do anything else' (Nightingale 1867, cited by Abel Smith 1960).

Good women were, and are, respectable and responsible. Skeggs (1997) explores how such responsibility is infused with the responsibility of class and nation. Good women have been presented as a civilising force within a nation and an empire. Skeggs quotes a mid-nineteenth century text on health and hygiene:

> The great means of improving the human race must be sought in the improvement of the health of woman, for she is the matrix in which the human statue is cast. Improve her health of body, of mind and of heart, and the human race would advance to perfection; deteriorate her, on the contrary, and in the same ration does it degenerate... In civilised nations matrons give the tone to society; for the rules of society are placed under their safeguard.
>
> (Tilt, 1852: 13, 261, cited in Skeggs 1997: 42)

Women are thus given both the responsibility for morality and the blame for its disruption. In nursing, as in other arenas, the 'higher class' of women were eventually established as the guardians and educators of the lower class nursing recruits as well as of the welfare of their patients. Skeggs' research on working-class women in further education identifies caring courses as continued mechanisms whereby 'young working-class women could be given responsibility (and encouraged to take pleasure) in the maintenance of social order... In this process they could also regulate themselves' (Skeggs 1997: 50).

It is women's role as mother that particularly emphasises the importance of women regulating themselves. As Kintz notes, 'while men are allowed to be both Boys and responsible Men, responsible women can only be Mothers' (Kintz 1996: 228). Images of female responsibility, however, derive from bourgeois notions of respectability.

'Good guy', citizen, gentleman

Similarly, in British society, responsible men appear to be seen as demonstrating a type of 'manliness' constructed through the public school system, a system in which sport plays a central role. (It is particularly through participation in and the enjoyment of sport that Men are still allowed to be Boys.) In the public schools

> true manliness was held to reside in the harmonious growth of the physique and the character side by side. A 'manly' boy was strong of body and pure of heart. The Victorian public school was the forcing-house of a new kind of masculinity in which the distinguishing characteristics of the male sex were not intellectual or genital but physical and moral. Man was neither a thinking machine nor was he governed by an unrestrained sexuality as animals were thought to be. He was loyal, brave, and active and as such a natural counterpart of woman who was spiritual, sensitive and vulnerable.
>
> (Holt 1989: 90)

The enemies of true manliness and sportsmanship were perceived as homosexuality and masturbation. Games were the means by which such activities were prevented, and sport was seen as a source of bodily purification and a celebration of what came to be known as 'muscular Christianity' (Holt 1989). The British love of games became an important hegemonic force, uniting different classes in a patriotism important in British imperial expansion. Among the middle classes, participation in sport fostered competition but also a sense of fair play; team spirit and leadership were qualities cultivated in the public schools, which saw themselves as developing the leaders of men and of empire. Physical strength and physical combat, such as pugilism, were, however, also strongly associated with working-class labour and pleasure. Sport allows manliness to accommodate both muscular physicality and qualities of courage, perseverance, discipline and co-operation.

If the 'good guy' is a sportsman and hence a team player, the 'gentleman' is also responsive to others. Gilmore concludes his cross cultural review of manhood by noting that

> manhood ideologies always include a criterion of selfless generosity, even to the point of sacrifice. Again and again we find that 'real' men are those who give more than they take; they love others... It is true that this male giving is different from, and less demonstrative and more obscure than, the female. It is less direct, less immediate, more involved with externals; the 'other' involved may be society in general, rather than specific persons.

> (Gilmore 1993: 229)

If real men are responsible, and responsible in the public sphere, they are, of course, leaders, politicians and managers. Men's public role is perhaps so taken for granted that the gendered nature of concepts such as citizenship has been ignored. Lister (1997) argues that the presumed universality of citizenship masks the exclusion of women from many of the rights and arenas of public life. Through feminist critiques of the theory and practice of citizenship, 'the universalist cloak of the abstract, disembodied individual has been cast aside to reveal a definitely male citizen and a white, heterosexual, non-disabled one at that' (Lister 1997: 66). Lister presents a dichotomy between public, male, citizen and private, female, non-citizen. Men are abstract thinkers, while women concentrate on the particular; men have a rational ability to apply dispassionate reason and standards of justice, while women are emotional and irrational; men are independent, active, heroic and strong, women are dependent, passive and weak; men uphold 'the realm of freedom', women maintain the 'realm of necessity' (p. 69).

Understandably, therefore, it is men who are the scientists, the lawyers, the judges, the doctors. When women adopt public leadership roles, they are mocked for their attention to detail, for being 'bossy' rather than bosses, and for their adherence to rules. Positive images of women as leaders are few. Margaret Thatcher was noted for being bossy and nannyish. Headmistresses and matrons are presented as dragons, vigilant in their guardianship of all within their realm.

'Bad guy': machismo masculinity

But men are not always responsible. On the contrary, masculinity can also represent reckless irresponsibility, dangerous and damaging aggression enacted through physical power and brutality, often combined with a protective territoriality apparently beyond the control of Kantian notions of reason. Connell (1993) has argued that a working-class hegemonic masculinity developed through industrialisation, emphasising physical strength and solidarity as a means of enabling working-class men to resist the power of managers and authoritarian fathers. As traditional male work roles decline and post-Fordist work practices result in an increase in casualised, often female, workers, more young men face structural unemployment. While academically able young men gain professional and managerial positions through education and training, others gain a sense of identity through masculinities characterised by chauvinism, machismo and toughness, associated with traditional worlds of manual labour (Willis 1977, Mac an Ghaill 1994). Unequal and, to some extent, oppositional masculinities develop.

Canaan (1996), in a study of the creative activities of young working-class men in Wolverhampton in the late 1980s, found a strong sense of local community and territory, used by the young men in her study to distinguish themselves from other similar localities and from middle-class people who occupied a 'different social and geographical location and set of values' (p. 118). Her subjects reported their enjoyment of drinking and fighting when asked about their creative activities. Drinking was linked to hardness and valued since loss of self-control often resulted in greater risk taking. Fighting involved not just physical control, but also careful observation and complex psychological awareness of self and others to distinguish between the 'hard' and those merely 'acting hard'. 'The quiet ones nearly always turn out to be the hardest' (Canaan 1996: 119). Fighting also served as a channel for displaced anger against those they were close to, or as a means of retribution for the emotional pain they may have inflicted on another. While young men saw females as pawns in their own game of power, older men sought more companionable relationships with women but nevertheless sought to protect their girlfriends from the potential danger from male drinking and fighting. Thus, assumptions about male dominance and female dependence persisted.

Canaan concludes that fighting and drinking involve both control and loss of control and thus lead to a repeated affirmation and loss of masculinity. When fighting, young men either asserted control over others or demonstrated their control over their own bodily pain; their indulgence in fighting to gain control stemmed from drinking that allowed them, paradoxically, to lose control. The tensions and contradictions inherent in such harsh, controlling, competitive, dominant, yet often excluded and subordinated masculinities, are present in constructions of antisocial male behaviour. The health effects of 'positive' and 'negative' masculinities are explored in Chapter 3.

Explaining masculinities and femininities

Early sociological explanations of the social constructions of masculinity and femininity concentrated on the congruence between gendered sets of attributes and the social roles that the majority of men and of women adopted in adult life. Socialisation into masculinity and femininity was functional for allocation into social roles. Interactionist approaches could explain the process of maintaining the social order through the perpetuation of meanings associated with symbols of masculinity and femininity. Feminist theorising exposed the limitations of such approaches, identifying the power of patriarchal assumptions that lay behind the constructions of femininity.

Understanding constructions of masculinity and femininity as part of broader ideological projects is a useful way of making visible the way in which assumptions about gender attributes support established social structures. The main ideological project is that of patriarchy. Patriarchy, however, is linked to a separate ideological project, the 'heterosexuality project'. As already indicated, the dominance of heterosexual assumptions within many of the gender constructions is visible by the way in which dominant masculinities and femininities have, hitherto, excluded gay men and lesbians. Homosexuality, however, currently constructs its own identities, sometimes through an appropriation of some of the icons of heterosexuality, such as muscularity (Champagne 1996, Smith 1996).

The control of sexuality is effected largely through what can be termed the 'morality project', whereby constructions of gender serve to maintain the moral order of society. Women bear the burden of the 'morality project'. Women's sexuality is controlled by ignoring women's own sexual needs and condemning those women who satisfy them. Sexual conquest for men is, in contrast, a valued attribute of some masculinities and contributes to the dominance of patriarchy. The morality project, however, entails more than the control of individual sexuality. It links with the heterosexuality project and to patriarchy and supports conventional notions of family life. Weeks (1991) attributes the introduction of Clause 28 into the Local Government Act 1986, which prohibited local authorities from 'promoting homosexuality', not so much to a reversal of the trend towards an acceptance of different sexualities but more to concern about the lack of a moral order accompanying diversity in family structures. Notions of family life retain a role in the maintenance of a moral order.

As already identified in Chapter 1, Marxist theory and dual systems theory would view gender constructions as inevitably linked to projects of economic and political power – the 'capitalism project'. Male work roles and women's domestic labour ultimately support the interests of the bourgeoisie. The 'gentleman' is not just part of the morality project but links morality to class and nation. Good women and gentlemen bore responsibility for the moral authority of the bourgeoisie and the dominant white race, for the honour of the nation, if not the empire.

The strength and importance of different social classes in the work sphere led, in Britain, to differing hegemonic masculinities: the manager, the bureaucrat, the entrepreneur, the boss, the 'Big Wheel', the manual worker who could sometimes be 'rough' but was usually 'respectable', the 'salt of the earth', the 'Sturdy Oak'. Those excluded from the successful economic enterprise could resort to deviant masculine identities as already indicated: bad guy, gangster, thug, hooligan – masculine cultures supported by health-threatening drinking and fighting.

The capitalism project can thus be seen as being supported by a range of subsidiary projects that individually and collectively support male dominance and thereby reinforce the patriarchal project. The management ideological project constructs views of entrepreneurial and organisational management that affect men and women at work (see Chapter 8). An accompanying political leadership project reinforces assumptions about men as leaders and, in sharing Enlightenment constructions of individual agency with the management project, maintains the dominance of a particular view of autonomous, instrumental (male) leadership. Men are leaders, women are led. Men's role as public figures is emphasised through male-gendered views of citizenship that illustrate how 'male' can be seen as synonymous with the person, privileging objectivity and offering service to the state. The service to the nation state, however, links to a further important project, the imperialist project, dependent on, in Britain, a complex mix of masculinities including public school notions of leadership, manliness, service and sportsmanship, coupled with notions of military service as officer (the officer as gentleman) or as soldier (the 'Sturdy Oak'). As Busfield notes, 'the ideal requirement for the conduct and characteristics of the military man constitute nigh on a roll call of idealised masculinity: bravery, courage, strength, endurance, discipline' (1996: 212).

Imperialism can be seen as being embedded in notions of hegemonic masculinity. White hegemonic masculinities excluded the experience of black men and constructed black masculinities as deviant. Early American theories of black masculinities deriving from functionalist standpoints constructed black males as absent from matrilineal family structures, black male loyalties as tribal and black male sexuality as pathologically excessive (Frazier 1966). More recently, black masculinities have been reanalysed as subordinated masculinity (Staples 1982, Mercer and Julien 1988), shaped through the oppressive structures of slavery that debarred black fathers from patriarchal privileges such as rights over children and access to paid employment. In this analysis, black males may, therefore, reject 'white' routes to employment and social position through education and the work ethic, adopting instead an excessive machismo or a committed hedonism.

The capitalist project could itself be seen as deriving from the Enlightenment project, which associated rationality with progress and viewed science as the epitome of objectivity. Objectivity and rationality were linked to masculinity, and thus gendered cultural codes are also implicated in what may be termed the 'knowledge project', that is, ideological assumptions that link men rather than women with publicly validated forms of knowledge. Rationality, in addition, links knowledge and gender to assumptions about autonomy and freedom, seen, in Enlightenment thought, as characteristics of a mature identity, more specifically of a mature male identity. Busfield notes the importance of rationality, autonomy, agency, power and gender in any analysis of constructions of gender and of mental health and mental disorder. Power is linked with rationality, and rationality with masculinity. Femininity is linked with irrationality and with 'the denial of agency'. Women lack the power to resist labelling as mentally ill (Busfield 1996: 108).

Recognising the links between assumptions about agency, forms of knowledge, gender and power, feminism has developed a feminist project that challenges the ideological assumptions inherent in constructions of masculinity and femininity. Feminist theories of knowledge have challenged the exclusion of emotions, feelings and personal experiences as valid sources of knowledge (see Chapter 9). Feminists have also challenged the separation of private and public spheres, seeking to understand how power structures affect their personal and public lives.

Bourdieu and cultural capital

The work of the French sociologist Pierre Bourdieu suggests ways of analysing cultural practices that provide a different way of understanding the diversity of masculinities and femininities as well as the distinctions made between genders. Bourdieu emphasises the importance of classification in social life. 'The social agents whom the sociologist classifies are producers not only of classifiable acts but also of acts of classification which are themselves classified' (Bourdieu 1986: 467). Thus, the social practice of individual men and women – 'a system of internalised embodied schemes' (p. 467) – are classifiable acts and acts of classification that are themselves classified.

The distinctions between masculinities (good guy/bad guy) and femininities (madonna/whore) and between masculinities and femininities are perpetuated because they are part of a collective history that is largely structured through the strength and movement of types of capital. Bourdieu emphasises the importance of cultural capital as well as economic capital. Individuals acquire and make use of both economic and cultural capital in their production of a meaningful world. Masculinities and femininities can, in themselves, be a source of cultural capital. Bourdieu argues that 'all the agents in a given social formation share a set of basic perceptual schemes', which derive ultimately from oppositions between the 'élite' and the 'mass' – high/low, spiritual/material, fine/coarse, light/heavy, free/forced, unique/ common, brilliant/dull. Fundamental oppositions (dominant/ dominated, temporal/spiritual, material/intellectual), Bourdieu suggests, support second, third or further oppositions, which can be traced back to fundamental relationships that express 'major relations of order' (high/low, strong/weak) associated with class-divided societies (p. 470). Thus, femininities and masculinities can become part of individuals' cultural capital, supporting divisions in the distribution of economic capital. Nevertheless, the fact that those who classify are also classified by those whom they classify means that dominant and dominated groups create their own judgments and distinctions about and between each other. Good women judge sexy nurses, who reject the values and criteria by which they are negatively judged. As Bourdieu notes,

The fact that in their relationship to the dominant classes, the dominated classes attribute to themselves strength in the sense of labour power and fighting strength – physical strength and also strength of character, courage, manliness – does not prevent the dominant groups from similarly conceiving the relationship in terms of the scheme strong/weak; but they reduce the strength which the dominated (or the young, or women) ascribe to themselves to brute strength, passion and instinct, a blind, unpredictable force of nature, the unreasoning violence of desire and they attribute to themselves spiritual and intellectual strength, a self-control that predisposes them to control others, a strength of soul or spirit which allows them to conceive their relationship to the dominated – the 'masses', women, the young – as that of the soul to the body, understanding to sensibility, culture to nature.

(p. 479)

Implicit in this extract from Bourdieu's detailed analysis of cultural distinctions is a clear view of the process of constructing positive and negative images of masculinity and femininity. The gentleman disapproves of the lout. The respectable women disapproves of the flirt. The practical nurse scorns the feminist intellectual. Nurses who seek to develop practical and caring skills alongside skills of analysis and decision making face conflicts that can only be understood through such cultural distinctions. Even the good woman is subordinated by her sensibility, her womanly nature and her care of the body.

Nursing gender, ideological projects and cultural capital

Representations of nursing draw on gender constructions that support broader ideological projects. 'Sexy nurse' is clearly supporting the heterosexual project as well as patriarchy. Male nurses, by definition, subvert masculinity by failing to conform to the 'No Sissy Stuff' dictum. Nurses, both male and female, are eroticised, seen as subordinate, giving and available. On the other hand, in nurse–client relationships there is the possibility for sexual exploitation on the part of the nurse. The possibility of such exploitation, however, is reduced through nurses' guardianship role in the morality project. Morality is seen to be safe with nurses. This brings nursing its own, albeit restricted, cultural capital. Nurses who transgress moral rules are deviant both as individuals and as nurses.

The low status of nursing tasks and care in a hierarchy of skill that privileges science and intellectual thought allows nursing to contribute passively to the 'knowledge project' by associating feminine cultural codes with the practical and emotional aspects of nursing. Nurses lack power in the political sphere, in management and in the economy through the intricacies of the way in which gendered constructions of knowledge, skill, leadership, management, power and autonomy reinforce the dominance of particular professional groups and support the interests of those who have economic capital. For nurses, gender and class interact to maintain nurses' subordinate position in contemporary industrialised societies (see Part II). Although British imperialist history can be seen as playing a significant role in the history of nursing, nurses' own role has been mythologised ('the lady with the lamp') rather than thoroughly explored, for example through looking at the contribution of nurses in the armed forces and military nurses within nursing. The contribution of Mary Seacole has been ignored for many decades. In so far as nursing history has been explored as part of the intellectual project of feminism, the story of male nurses has yet to be told.

Analysing gender constructions as ideological projects, or as aspects of cultural capital, however, is part of an analytical tradition that has been criticised through discourses of postmodernism. It is possible that gendered images are framed through discourses that are becoming more loosely connected to social structures and more obviously malleable. Individual nurses, in so far as they both recognise and reject the constructions of gender presented here and the stereotypical responses that they encounter in their daily lives, inevitably deconstruct and reconstruct gendered practices. Indeed, nurses, it can be argued, are used within media constructions to subvert (but not too dangerously) the 'natural' order of the world. It is interesting how, in the television programme *Casualty*, a male nurse marries a female doctor and black male nurses have relationships with white women who are managers or doctors, subverting not only the inferiority of their subordinate class position, but also the subordination of their race. If black men are sexual predators and dangerous to hegemonic white masculinity, the danger is curiously neutralised when the black male is a nurse – further proof that the morality project is safe with nurses. Therein lies nurses' strength in gender reconstruction and dissolution. Nurses have opportunities to shape masculinities and femininities in ways that challenge dominant groups' conceptions of the dominant/dominated order. It is not in nurses' interests to maintain distinctions between the soul and the body, understanding and sensibility, culture and nature (Bourdieu 1986: 479). Nor, as Chapter 3 demonstrates, is it in the interests of our collective health.

3   Gender and health

Introduction

Gender differences in health and illness can be succinctly summarised in the phrase 'women get sicker but men die quicker'. Life expectancy is longer for women than for men, yet women perceive themselves as being less healthy and use health services more frequently than men (Miles 1991, Doyal 1995, Macintyre *et al.* 1996). Men and women differ in their health care practices: whereas men tend not to talk about their health and are reluctant to change health-threatening behaviour, women are perceived as being more willing to discuss health in the context of their lives. This chapter looks briefly but critically at the evidence for the general view that mortality rates are higher among men and morbidity rates higher among women, and then looks at different explanations for gender differences in health. Changes in social structure and the diversity of masculinities and femininities ensure that the relationship between gender and health is a changing one, dependent on an individual life course within a changing sociocultural system. Nevertheless, features of the gender order – roles in the labour market, sexual relationships and power relationships between men and women – influence gender and health. This chapter explores the way in which masculinity and femininity as cultural scripts can have a protective or damaging effect on health.

Mortality rates

Male life expectancy is less than that of women in all but a few Asian countries (Doyal 1995). In Western countries, the male mortality disadvantage was relatively small at the beginning of the twentieth century. However, female mortality fell more rapidly than male until, by 1979, females in the United States had a relative advantage of 7.8 years (Waldron 1995). The gap between male and female mortality rates in Western societies has begun to narrow during the 1980s and 90s; cultural trends and their effects on men and women are not static. The 1998 government Independent Inquiry into Inequalities in Health, chaired by Sir Donald Acheson, reports that, in Britain, 'in 1971 males had a 64 per cent higher mortality rate than women. By 1996 this had reduced to a 55 per cent higher rate in men' (Acheson 1998: 101). Gender differences in mortality rate are particularly pronounced in youth and early adulthood. By the age of 15, boys have a 65 per cent higher mortality than girls (Botting 1997) and between 20 and 24 years, the mortality rate for men is 2.8 times higher than that for women (Dunnell 1991, Tickle 1996). In Britain, life expectancy for women is five years longer than for men, although the gap is beginning to narrow (Acheson 1998, ONS 1998a).

The main causes of lower life expectancy for men lie in higher deaths rates for coronary heart disease, lung cancer and chronic obstructive airways disease, accidents, homicides, suicides and AIDS. The higher rates are normally explained by reference to differences between men's and women's lifestyles. Occupational hazards resulting in airways disease and deaths through accidents have affected men more than women. Cigarette smoking has, hitherto, been a major cause of male death. It is only in the 1990s that women's rate of smoking has been similar to men's (ONS 1999). Men drink more than women, and alcohol-related deaths, including those in motor vehicle accidents, account for some excess deaths. Suicide among men has increased in recent years, particularly among young men, but accidents and homicides have always been a feature of masculine rather than feminine behaviour. Men also meet death through physical risk taking more frequently than women. Men's life-threatening risk taking behaviour includes drug taking and addiction, but men's higher level of exercise participation may counteract some of the health disadvantages apparently resulting from men's lifestyles (ONS 1997, Acheson 1998).

Trends that are reducing the gap between male and female death rates include women's increased participation in driving. Although there are decreasing gender differences in the amount of driving, however, there are increasing differences in driving-related safety. In the United States, for example, women have increased their use of seat belts more than men and reduced their driving-related alcohol consumption (Piani and Schoenborn 1993, Waldron 1995). Although young women, but not young men, of school age have increased their cigarette consumption (ONS 1999), in Britain and the United States females are not increasingly adopting a broad range of risky behaviours (Waldron 1995, Acheson 1998).

Morbidity

It is women who appear to feel less healthy than men. Blaxter's study of health and lifestyles reports that when asked to think of a person they thought of as healthy, of those who could think of someone (and almost 15 per cent could not), 80 per cent of males and 57 per cent of females mentioned a man. Women, however, gave more complex and expansive answers to questions about health than men and were considerably more likely to define health in terms of social relationships (Blaxter 1990). In Britain, data from the 1994 General Household Survey showed a higher rate of disability among women than among men; healthy life expectancy for women is only two or three years greater than for men (Acheson 1998).

Women are widely reported as suffering from more mental disorder than men. Doyal notes that in 'community services throughout the developed world, women report about twice as much anxiety and depression as men' (Doyal 1995: 11). Busfield reports that US and UK surveys of psychiatric disorder in the community usually show twice as many female as male sufferers (Busfield 1996: 14). There are, however, distinctive gender patterns associated with different mental phenomena. While anorexia nervosa is a predominantly female condition and women report rates for anxiety, phobias and depression twice those of men, diagnoses of schizophrenia, paranoia or mania do not show a gender preference, and substance use disorders are more common among men than women (Meltzer *et al.* 1995, Busfield 1996).

A difficulty in assessing morbidity is that of separating factors affecting the reporting of a condition from factors affecting the condition itself. Women are higher users of health services than men, but the reasons for this are difficult to unravel. Women live longer, and use of the health service increases with age. Higher consultation rates over a lifetime would therefore be expected, especially taking into account the necessary health service contact prompted by the normal processes of pregnancy and childbirth. Furthermore, women appear to find it easier to discuss their own health and may find it more socially acceptable to do so (Blaxter 1990).

Methodological difficulties involved in studying gender and health

The possible gender bias involved in the reporting of morbidity is only one of the methodological difficulties involved in researching gender and health. A problem with identifying the effects of any social or cultural factors is that death may be classified by the proximate cause, without acknowledging distal factors that may have had a progressive influence on ill health and may have been affected by lifestyle and the effects of gender on social status. In addition, the effects of other dimensions of inequality, particularly socio-economic position, are difficult to separate from the effects of gender. Furthermore, the fact that gender is a cultural construction that is embedded in social life means that gendered assumptions about the world may affect the questions we ask about the relationship between social factors and health, as well as the answers we provide. Doyal (1995) suggests that the lack of female influence on the allocation of funds for medical research may have resulted in the lack of research into conditions such as osteoporosis and incontinence, which affect mainly women. Doyal also notes, as do other writers (Lorber 1997), that research into coronary heart disease has been carried out on men but not on women, on the problematic assumption that there would be no difference between a male and female response to disease or treatment. Bias also occurs through the way in which conditions are defined. This is most obviously the case with mental health, but 'because illness is socially constructed, physicians and patients may see the same set of symptoms (or lack of them) entirely differently' (Lorber 1997: 4).

Gendered assumptions and gender differences in social processes may also affect the measures used to study morbidity. If morbidity is measured by days off work, by contact with health care services, by medication use or by self-reporting measures, gender variations in patterns of work, in responsibilities for others, in the willingness to acknowledge and attend to minor symptoms, will all affect the measures, making it difficult to separate an account of health differences from cultural constructions of gender and cultural constructions of health. Too easy an acceptance on the part of researchers that 'men die quicker and women get sicker' can lead to the construction of research studies that seek confirming data rather than attempting an objective review. An interest in women's psychological morbidity resulting from their social roles, for example, can lead to asking different questions about women from those asked about men. Annandale notes that

> studies of women may stress social support at work, and the possibility of conflict between 'home and work', while research on men's health might attend to physical hazards to health obviating the possibility of looking at the interlacing of 'family and work' for men, and effectively denying the real dangers that women experience in the workplace (which includes the home).
>
> (1998a: 121)

Even more significant, perhaps, is the apparent failure of researchers to report similarities rather than differences between men's and women's reporting of health and ill health. Macintyre *et al.* (1996), in a report on their analyses of two British studies, the Health and Lifestyles Survey and the West of Scotland Twenty-07 study, found that the rates of longstanding illness were the same for men and for women; women's higher rate of symptom reporting was only consistent across the life span for psychological manifestations of distress. Gender differences were apparent for specific illnesses at different ages, rheumatoid arthritis being more common in older females and asthma more common in younger males.

Researchers' stress on women's ill health may be explicable by the feminist standpoint adopted by many of the researchers (discussed below). Two studies that have, however, attempted to determine whether women do experience more ill health, rather than simply report more symptoms, than men; both conclude that women are not over-reporting illness. Annandale (1998b) refers to Davis's (1981) study of chronic joint symptoms associated with osteoarthritis and Macintyre's (1993) study of the common cold. Both of these studies used 'objective' measures to measure the severity of symptoms. Radiographic evidence was graded by two rheumatologists in Davis's study, and clinical observers recorded the presence or absence of a cold and its severity in Macintyre's study. Both studies found no evidence of women over-reporting symptoms; on the contrary, men appeared to rate their pain and symptoms more severely than women. Annandale (1998b) advises caution in identifying gender differences in health behaviour and experience of health and illness.

Explaining gender differences in health

Early sociological explanations for gender differences in mortality and morbidity concentrated on the differences between men's and women's social roles, particularly their roles in the domestic and paid division of labour. Analyses based on a gender division of labour at home and at work suggest that the excess of male premature mortality is due to the fact 'that males live in a much more dangerous world than do females' (Stillion 1995: 50). They have considerably higher accident, suicide and homicide rates than females. Higher accident rates derive from both external factors such as workplace conditions and from an internal readiness, willingness and skill to avoid or deal with external situations that threaten safety. The necessity for men to remain in health-threatening work situations and to participate in risk taking behaviour can be seen, from a functionalist standpoint, to be part of the male role in a society in which it is men who take the responsibility for providing for the economic wellbeing of the family. As we have already seen, male roles are supported by the cultural construction of masculinities as the 'Big Wheel', the 'Sturdy Oak', able to 'Give 'em Hell'.

If men are the providers, it is women who are provided for, while they labour in the home. Chesler (1972) argued that the way in which behaviour is defined and interpreted is central to the attribution of mental disorder, noting that departures from sex-role expectations are defined as signs of mental disorder. There is a 'Catch 22' for women: 'both close conformity to, and departure from, female roles are liable to generate definitions of psychiatric disorder' (Busfield 1996: 101). Women obsessive about, and women neglectful of, domestic tasks have both been at risk of being labelled as mentally ill. Feminine role behaviour can also be seen as more closely allied to 'sick role' behaviour. Both assume dependency and compliance, making it easier for women to consult a doctor, thus accounting for the higher consultation rate among women than men (Balint *et al.* 1970, Oakley 1976).

Gove and Tudor (1973) found that women's higher incidence of mental illness could be attributable to their social situation. Through an extensive review of the evidence on male and female mortality and morbidity in America from 1945 to 1970, it appeared that it was not the general expectations of the feminine role that induced symptoms, but the specific expectations and obligations of marriage. Married women were often restricted to housewifery, an unstructured, boring, frustrating activity with time to brood over troubles and to notice signs of ill health (Gove and Tudor 1973, Miers 1979). Even when working, married women may experience frustration through employment in roles not commensurate with their educational background and may experience the stress of multiple roles as mother, worker and wife. Conflicting and diffuse social expectations were seen as bringing mental costs. Oakley (1974) found that 70 per cent of housewives in her study of housework were dissatisfied with the job of housework, attributing mental health costs to the isolation, loneliness and monotony of the work. Women's caring obligations, however, may be protective of health: responsibility for others may restrict women's willingness to indulge in risk taking behaviour.

Women, work and health

Whether or not work outside the home brings health gains for women, or further stresses through role conflict, has been extensively, if inconclusively, explored (Arber *et al.* 1985, Bartley *et al.* 1992). The benefits of paid work appear to include financial rewards, social support and self-esteem, but work outside the home can result in long hours of domestic and paid labour. As Doyal notes, however, 'neither "women" nor "work" are homogenous categories' (1995: 155). Studies exploring the effects of household composition, age, division of labour in the home, hours worked and nature of employment have revealed the complexity of the variables that affect employed women's health

(Arber *et al.* 1985). Bartley *et al.* (1992) found some evidence of part-time, but not full-time, work benefitting the health of women with young children, although women in the highest income group appeared to benefit from full-time work. Overall, psychological gains seemed to be greater than physical benefits. Studies of health and unemployment among males suggest that a lack of paid work may affect men's and women's health in a similar way (Bartley 1994). Psychological costs may be similar, and, for both men and women, paid work may bring the greatest health benefit to those on lowest incomes.

Socio-economic position and gender differences in health

Attempts to determine how socio-economic status interacts with gender in affecting health are hindered by the difficulties of devising adequate measures of socio-economic position for women. Using the husband's or father's occupation as the basis for assigning women to a social class has been regarded as inadequate for several decades, but assigning social class position to a woman on the basis of her current occupation also poses difficulties. The Registrar General's classification is based on a male occupational structure and relies on traditional assumptions about the importance of occupations that do not adequately reflect the range of work that women do. As a result, 'about two-thirds of women in paid work end up coded as Social Class III non-manual (for example secretaries, shop assistants, clerical workers) and to a lesser extent as Class II (for example teachers, nurses)' (Annandale 1998b: 149). Hence, observing class gradients in women's health is difficult. Government changes to social class classification will address this issue. Arber (1990), in a review of General Household Survey data, demonstrated that 'to understand women's health status it is important to analyse simultaneously occupational class, marital roles and employment status' (p. 52). More recently, she has suggested that more attention should be given to educational qualifications in health inequalities research as education influences both occupational class and employment status (Arber 1997).

Research into the effects of caring roles, paid or unpaid, on health, presents a complex picture. Analyses of data from the 1985 and 1990 General Household Surveys demonstrate that unpaid caring has economic consequences, affecting employment opportunities and resulting in lower family net income in comparison with non-carers. The self-reported health of unpaid carers was similar to that of non-carers, although caring for over 50 hours a week, caring co-residentially, caring for someone on one's own and caring for someone with physical and mental impairments were associated with less good health (Evandrou 1996: 226). Informal carers caring for someone outside their own home, however, were more likely to report good health than non-carers, suggesting that caring does not, in itself, necessarily have a negative effect on health and that wellbeing may be more easily maintained in more distant relationships between carer and cared for. Doyal (1995), however, has summarised some of the health risks for nurses at their place of work, including accidents, injury, toxic chemicals, radiation and stress. Nolan and Grant (1992), in a study of a sample of carers drawn from the National Carers Association, found that carers combined high levels of stress with high levels of satisfaction.

Research concerning socio-economic factors and health has begun to identify health differentials within social class groupings as well as between them and to look at dimensions of the psychosocial work environment as well as the influence of supportive social networks in communities. Marmot and Feeney (1996), for example, have looked at the effects of 'work demands', 'control' and 'support at work' on health in the work setting, finding that a higher degree of control was associated with better health, and a low degree of control associated with poorer health. The Acheson Report takes seriously the argument that good social networks are health enhancing (Acheson 1998). The intricacies of demands, control and support may be the mechanisms that link social status to health through biological processes of stress response.

There is considerable evidence, however, for the view that women's different occupational and domestic positions make them more vulnerable to poverty than men throughout their life course. Women are more likely to work part time in low-paid work and to have breaks in employment, thus making them less likely than men to be eligible for contributory state benefits and more likely to be dependent on Income Support (Lister 1992, DSS 1997). Concern for the health consequences for poorer families has led to recommendations for policies that will reduce the psychosocial ill health of young women in disadvantaged circumstances (Acheson 1998).

The Health and Lifestyle Survey showed that women with children under the age of five were most likely to show signs of psychological ill health (Blaxter 1990). Material disadvantage is strongly related to stress-related conditions such as anxiety, depression and migraine in mothers with young children (Graham 1993, Baker and Taylor 1997, Brown and Harris 1978) as well as to health-damaging behaviour such as smoking (Graham 1987). A further recommendation in the Acheson Report is to seek policies that reduce disability and ameliorate its consequences in older women, particularly those living alone. Again, it is older women more than older men whose quality of life is reduced by low income, which, coupled with the extra expense of being more likely to live alone, puts them at risk of, for example, 'fuel poverty'.

Feminism, gender and health

Feminist approaches to the study of health and illness posed a major challenge to functionalist, Marxist and interactionist sociologies from the 1970s onwards. Liberal feminism may be seen as having limited influence on an understanding of gender and health since it promotes what Annandale sees as an assimilationist agenda, viewing women as similar to men through accepting the rationalist privileging of 'mind' over 'body'. Patriarchy works, in the liberal feminist view, through excluding women from valued social statuses and social spheres (Annandale 1998a, 1998b). Liberal feminism fails to recognise the way in which concepts of rationality themselves both depend on and support the patriarchal project through associating men with rationality and agency and women with irrationality and passivity. Busfield has argued that

> Gender is indirectly embedded in the formal constructions of mental disorder. This is because, although formally described in universal terms, the characteristics of specific disorders refer to mental life and behaviour that is to a greater or lesser extent gendered (and also specific to class and ethnicity)... For example, to the extent that fear, anxiety and sadness are deemed more appropriate, reasonable feelings in women than in men, then the categories of disorder constructed around pathologies of these feelings will end up identifying more female than male disturbance.
>
> (1996: 103)

Busfield notes that assumptions about normality, maturity, agency and rationality construct mental disorder as exemplifying a lack of agency and rationality. Mental disorder is 'a world in which individuals are assumed to be subject to forces which they themselves cannot immediately control – they are passive rather than active' (p. 105). These contrasts are linked to gender because the passive/active opposition is at the core of cultural constructions of femininity and masculinity.

Annandale (1998b) notes that liberal feminism's strong emphasis on the health disadvantages for women of domestic labour and the housewife role led to assumptions about the importance of the public as opposed to the private sphere. This in itself devalued the lives of many women, leading eventually to strong critiques of feminism for its middle-class-dominated agendas, which failed to recognise and valorise the diversity of women's experience.

In contrast, radical feminism saw patriarchy as controlling women's health through controlling women's bodies. From this standpoint, the medical profession is complicit in the control of women. Medical language constructs women as objects to be degraded and manipulated. Daly (1979) notes the use of gynaeco-logical terms such as 'incompetent cervix'. The solution is for women to take control of their own bodies and their own health, celebrating women's experience of their bodies and women's natural biological processes such as procreation. Radical feminists have explored the constraining and enabling potential of new reproductive technologies and paid close attention to childbirth (Stanworth 1987).

Materialist feminisms focus on the health effects of economic circumstances of women brought about through the development of capitalist societies. Writers who have concentrated on exploring women's oppression through labour market processes have, however, made little explicit reference to health. There is now a growing emphasis on identifying the health hazards of women's paid and unpaid work (Doyal 1995).

Gender, cultural codes and health

While acknowledging the contribution of feminism to an understanding of gender and health, Annandale (1998b) argues that the dichotomous category of male/female 'blinds us to the heterogeneity and plurality of experience that characterises contemporary social life' (p. 153). She suggests that the opposition between men and women links to the opposition between health and disease, leading to a patriarchal construction of men as healthy and women as unhealthy. A search for a new approach has led Annandale to an exploration of links between health and different constructions of masculinity and femininity, an approach I adopt. Annandale and Hunt (1990) used the Bem Sex Role Inventory (Bem 1974) to study the relationship between sex-role orientation and self-reported health. The 'masculinity' and 'femininity' scores were more significant than male or female sex as a variable. High masculinity scores were associated with better health for both men and women. An exploration of the links between health and differing cultural constructions of masculinity and femininity may help to illuminate similarity and diversity within and across genders while still acknowledging the influence of the ideological projects that permeate and construct our gendered culture.

Measuring masculinity

Studying the relationship between masculinity and health has led to a distinction between positive and negative masculinity. The Bem Sex Role Inventory (Bem 1974) and a similar Personal Attributes Questionnaire (Spence *et al.* 1974) both use masculinity scales that reflect perceptions of desirable characteristics of masculinity such as agency and self-confidence. Such characteristics are associated with health for both men and women. In 1979, Spence *et al.* extended the Personal Attributes Questionnaire to include an additional masculinity scale reflecting the negative aspects of masculinity. As Helgeson (1995) explains, 'self-confident is an item on the positive masculinity scale... and arrogant is an item on the negative masculinity scale' (p. 70). The two scales are positively correlated, however, suggesting agency as an underlying linking dimension. Characteristics of masculinity perceived as desirable have been termed 'trait masculinity'.

A different approach has been to study aspects of male gender role that are sources of stress or conflict. The Masculine Gender Role Stress Scale identifies sources of stress for males because of conflict with hegemonic notions of masculinity. These sources of stress are physical inadequacy, emotional inexpressiveness, subordination to women, intellectual inferiority and performance failure (Eisler and Skidmore 1987). Helgeson (1995) notes that other scales developed along similar lines reflect four themes: success, power and competition; restrictive emotionality; restrictive affectionate behaviour between men; and conflicts between work and family relations. The sources of role conflict are seen as 'fear of femininity' (Helgeson 1995: 70). Yet more scales focus on men's perceptions of how men ought to behave (Brannon and Juni 1984, Pleck *et al.* 1993).

Masculinity and health

Trait masculinity has been widely reported as having a positive effect on the psychological wellbeing of both men and women (Whitley 1984, Annandale and Hunt 1990, Helgeson 1995), particularly in terms of reduced depression, reduced anxiety and enhanced self-esteem. (It is interesting to note that although many women may demonstrate confidence and control, this is not necessarily an expectation of femininity.) Negative masculinity scales and the role stress scales and role conflict scales, on the other hand, are linked to lower psychological wellbeing (Helgeson 1995). These more negative measures of masculinity appear to be related to risk producing behaviour such as smoking, alcohol use and poor dietary and exercise habits (Eisler *et al.* 1988).

Despite the link between positive health and trait masculinity scores, however, there is substantial research evidence that links attributes of masculinity to the risk of coronary heart disease. Details of the research cannot be discussed here, but it is worth noting that the most lethal components of the behaviour patterns studied – hostility and time urgency – are linked to negative masculinity scores. High negative masculinity scores were linked to a long time interval between first noticing warning signs and the development of an acute myocardial condition. Negative masculinity predicted more severe heart attacks. Positive masculinity predicted a greater degree of social support. Empathy and a lack of homophobia predicted the presence of a confidant (Helgeson 1995: 84). The finding that negative masculinity can be distinguished from positive masculinity is, however, important. Negative masculinity seems to be linked to poor social networks and poor health. Positive masculinity may be positively linked to health.

Masculine role stress and role conflict measures suggest that 'fear of femininity' puts men at a disadvantage in terms of health-supporting measures such as social support, and close emotional relationships. Helgeson cites an extensive list of research studies indicating that a lack of social support is linked to mortality (Blazer 1982, House *et al.* 1982) and suggest that the male emphasis on detachment and objectivity may inhibit close relationships. A male repression of emotion may also have health consequences (Pennebaker *et al.* 1988). A study of empathy and social support (Trobst *et al.* 1994) has shown that differences between men's and women's social support can be accounted for by women's greater empathy. A lack of empathy may be associated with a lack of attention to feelings and emotions of self and others, which can lead to a lack of attention to symptoms. Men's relationships with men are often orientated towards activity rather than feelings, which may place men at a support disadvantage. However, men's friendships may involve informational and instrumental support, features consistent with masculinity.

Masculinities, femininities and health

Whereas many positive masculinities, for example 'gentleman', 'citizen' and 'leader', may have positive effects on health, negative masculinities have negative health consequences for men and also for women. Male violence to each other and to women is a health problem. Doyal (1995) describes domestic violence as a public health issue on a global scale (p. 53). Busfield (1996) notes the long-term effects of sexual abuse in terms of anxiety, anger, hostility and depression. She notes that it is feelings of powerlessness that help to determine the meanings attached to events and their long-term consequences. The association between women and ill health may derive from associations between femininity, and passivity and powerlessness. The negative associations between femininity and ill health may, however, derive from psychoanalytic explanations for women's lack of psychological wellbeing. These, in various ways, construct a view of women's neediness that derives from the expectations placed upon a young girl to defer to others and to be connected to others as part of the development of self (see Chapter 7). Such neediness results in anxiety and dependence, placing women at risk of the sometimes abusive power of male control.

Masculinity, it could be argued, has constructed a femininity that cannot challenge male control over the positive, health-enhancing attributes of control and self-confidence. Women who take control with confidence are often perceived negatively, being described as 'bossy' and, in nursing, being perceived as 'battle-axe' or 'dragon'. Masculinity has also denied femininity a sense of value, other than through the idealisation of motherhood, a process that allows the health-enhancing attributes of a mother's support to be taken for granted and unacknowledged. If femininity is devalued, it is to be feared, and masculinity, be it positive or negative, cannot acknowledge any shared characteristics with the 'good woman'. Horrocks (1994), writing from his experience as a psychotherapist, identifies what he calls the cryptic message of masculinity:

> don't accept who you are. Conceal your weakness, your tears, your fear of death, your love for others. Conceal your impotence. Conceal your potency. Disparage women since they remind you too much of your feminine side. Disparage gay men since that's too near the bone as well. Fake your behaviour. Dominate others, then you can fool everyone, especially yourself, that you feel powerful.
>
> (p. 25)

Horrocks argues that patriarchy has damaged men as it has damaged women, and that feminisms, in valorising women, disparage men. Acknowledging the diversity within both masculinities and femininities – as well as valorising the identities of individual men and women – may help to identify similarities between positive trait masculinity and the health-protective characteristics of the 'good woman'. Although mothers are taken for granted, mothers as good women are noticed for their responsibility, their respectability and their concern for others. These are health-protective characteristics, rigorously inhibiting risk taking behaviour and their associated health costs. The agentic self-control implicit in such femininities is curiously invisible in the active/passive construction of men and women, but so too is the other-orientation implicit in the responsibility of men's public roles. Deconstructing gendered assumptions may lead to interesting lines of enquiry in relation to gender and health. Is confident femininity health enhancing?

Such discussions can appear to ignore the importance of the socio-economic conditions already alluded to, which differentially affect the health of men and women as well as of their families. However, the fact that researchers concerned with inequalities in health are currently exploring the importance of psychosocial factors and of social support as explanatory variables is important. Such developments occur at a time when the health costs of controlling, negative masculinity (which may or may not be founded on a fear of femininity) are encouraging health care practitioners to take both men's and women's health seriously. This involves taking the cultural construction of gender seriously. For health care practitioners, it involves taking one's own assumptions about gender seriously enough to subject them to critical yet empathetic scrutiny.

Gendered assumptions about men and women, sometimes deriving from accurate data on overall gender differences in mortality and morbidity, can have a significant effect on treatment. Lorber (1997) notes that women with symptoms of heart disease in the United States receive less active treatment than men, with significant adverse consequences (Wenger 1994). Furthermore, women consulting women physicians have been shown to be more likely to have had a cervical smear test or a mammogram than women with male physicians (Franks and Clancy 1993). Writers concerned with men's health studies are now identifying the difficulties that men have in engaging with preventive health services. Health promotion, for example, can appear a gendered concern – a concern for women, not men. Cameron and Bernardes (1998) noted that among their sample of men who had contacted the Prostate Help Association, there were some who had ignored their symptoms for many years. Nurses who understand the construction of femininities and masculinities will help men and women with diverse gender identities to receive flexible, reflective and responsive health care. Nursing is so closely associated with women that gender will always be an issue for nurses. The following chapters explore the influence of cultural constructions of gender on the development of nursing and the understanding of nurses' work.

PART II

Gender and nursing

4 Choosing to nurse: from Florence Nightingale to the National Health Service

Introduction

This chapter looks at the influence of cultural constructions of masculinity and femininity both on the development of nursing as a profession and on nursing recruitment. It concentrates on the influence of nineteenth and early twentieth century views of middle-class femininity. A review of the development of nursing through the Crimean war is followed by a review of men in nursing in the nineteenth century. The chapter concludes by looking at changes in nursing and health care from 1900 to 1945. The role of nurses and women in the 'morality project', identified in Chapter 2, becomes clear.

The preponderance of women in nursing makes it seem as though gender must be an important factor in choosing to nurse. As noted in the 1972 Report of the Committee on Nursing, the necessity for national recruitment campaigns to emphasise the changing and diverse nature of nursing stems from 'the prevalence of a strong feeling, not least among nurses and midwives, that nurses and midwives are "born not made", perhaps the most stubborn of all the stereotypes' (Briggs 1972: 31). Such an essentialist view of nursing is supported by, and supportive of, a strong nursing tradition among families, leading, at the time of the Briggs Report, to a concern that nursing and midwifery were not considered seriously by young people lacking close connections to the profession. It is, however, generally girls who are seen as 'born nurses', reflecting an essentialist view of both nursing and gender. A functionalist, sex-role analysis, privileging the importance of motherhood and associated caring attributes, can also be drawn upon to explain the view that nursing is women's work. Essentialist and functionalist views of gender differences, however, ignore the influence of the range of ideological projects identified in Chapter 2. Acknowledging gender as a cultural construction that is both diverse and changing over time allows us to see that choosing to nurse can be seen as a different experience for men and women from different backgrounds, in different social circumstances and at different historical epochs.

Images of nursing, however, draw heavily on particular accounts of nursing's history, sustained through what the Briggs Report identifies as 'the inherited image of the hospital nurse' (Briggs 1972: 23). Features of this image include the linking of doctors and nurses not as partners but 'as people in charge on one hand and their "handmaidens" on the other'; the recognition that sex differences between doctors and nurses provide 'the essence of the drama' in relationships that can involve friction; and a class element linking vocation with Nightingale's 'higher class of woman' and the enforcement of the discipline of a vocation through matron's hierarchical control (Briggs 1972: 23–4).

The Briggs Report suggested that the twentieth century mass media is responsible for the sustained power of nineteenth century images of nursing. Romantic literature and popular women's magazines as well as television series and films has created a separate hospital world with its own dramas, spotlighting the romantic relationships of nurses with both doctors and patients. Newspaper reporting on nursing, although frequent, has often been of a fragmented and personalised nature (Briggs 1972: 27).

Even in the educational press, at the end of the century, as I have noted in a review of coverage of nursing issues in *The Times Higher Educational Supplement* (now *The Higher*), 'most photographic images of nurses and of nursing are disappointingly stereotypical, framed within a medical model, with female nurses, frilly hats and hospital equipment illustrating articles which focus on change' (Miers, 1996: 20). Thus, despite the changing cultural constructions of gender, cultural constructions of nursing appear to emphasise continuity in both relationships within health care and relationships between men and women. Understandably, therefore, if nursing is a natural job for women, it is not surprising that there are few studies concerning why women choose to nurse. The limited literature on men in nursing, discussed more fully in

Chapter 5, focuses on men's career progression rather than their choice of nursing as a career (Milligan 1993).

If both nursing and gender are cultural constructions, the reasons why men and women may enter nursing and the extent to which cultural assumptions about gender affect individual decisions need to be considered in terms of the dominant constructions of femininity and masculinity in different historical periods. There is, however, no one history of femininity and masculinity, nor one history of nursing, but only histories, written from the standpoints of different decades and through different assumptions.

Nursing in the nineteenth century

Davies (1980) has identified the influence of a 'history as progress' view on nursing history leading to an emphasis on the heroic achievements of exceptional individuals. Her edited collection of essays, *Rewriting Nursing History*, begins with pictorial representations of nursing's progress during the nineteenth century. It is a representation of the progress from Sarah Gamp to ministering angel. As Davies notes:

> The old, wrinkled, fat character looks away from us, a sure sign of a shifty and unreliable person. She is bleary-eyed and the cause of her obvious preoccupation is something on which one would hesitate to enquire. The attractive, pure and unsullied-looking woman, the new modern nurse, holds our gaze in a calm and coolly attentive way. There is a cross behind her, not a bottle and a gamp.
>
> (1980: 11)

The sign of nursing progress (from 1838 to 1888) is the difference between a rough disreputable woman of the lower classes and the virtue and respectability of youthful, middle-class femininity. Health care in the nineteenth century would have been provided in the home, either by members of the household, particularly women, or through the paid services of medical men (qualified practitioners or attendants), a 'private nurse' or a 'handy-woman'. For many middle-class families with domestic servants, it would be the servants who would be charged with the task of caring for the sick, but if this were not possible, additional labour would be bought in. The household income determined the nature of the additional labour; households with more income would be better able to select women of sensibility and respectability (private nurses) for the duties typical of handy-women, working-class women able to take charge of the care of the sick, childbirth and laying out of the dead. Additionally, health care could be provided through voluntary hospitals, which were supported by charitable donations and by individual payments, or through institutions provided through the Poor Law.

Handy-women and private nurses

'Handy-women' became, as Dingwall *et al.* (1988) note, 'probably the largest group of paid carers operating throughout the nineteenth century and well into the twentieth' (p. 9). In the Poor Law workhouses, direct care would have been provided by 'pauper nurses', those who could not get employment elsewhere. Poor women thus provided services to other poor women. Not-so-poor women provided services to their social superiors. The difference between the handy-woman and the private nurse can be seen as the difference between rough, impoverished femininity and the respectability deemed suitable by the middle class. Women working as private nurses in middle-class households held a status similar to, but more specialised than, that of a servant. Maggs (1986) has noted the uncertainty of the status of young women employed as private nurses, leading to fictionalised accounts of romantic intrigue between private nurses and sons of the household in late Victorian times (Dingwall *et al.* 1988). The 1950s and 60s' emphasis on nursing as a romantic and upwardly mobile career choice for young women, portrayed through television series such as *Emergency Ward 10* and *Dr Kildare*, may thus have a long history.

Dingwall *et al.* (1988: 16) note that although it is unhelpful to draw a clear distinction between a handywoman and a private nurse,

the social distinctions are important: private nurses were integrated into the service of the affluent while handywomen were autonomous workers among the poor. Private nurses were likely to command other servants while handywomen laboured on their own or in partnership with other members of the family.

These different roles and relationships within the household were mirrored by differences between the ordinary nurses and sisters and matrons employed within workhouses and voluntary hospitals. The qualities seen necessary for senior hospital nurses were those of the respectable 'good woman', as an advertisement in 1852 for a post as matron at Leeds General Infirmary illustrates. Candidates were required to be

> staid, sober and discreet, mild and humane disposition, at the same time possessed of firmness to rule the household; it is also desirable that she be experienced in the management of a family and the duties of a sick room.
>
> (Woodward 1974: 30, cited in Dingwall *et al.* 1988: 16)

The 'history as progress' view of nursing development suggests that it was the development of medical knowledge that led to the increasing importance of hospitals. Hospitals became places for careful observation and experimentation in treatment, which led to improved medical care. For medical knowledge to develop, doctors had to rely on the reliability and quality of nurses' assistance in observation and treatment. Furthermore, as treatments became effective, more and more higher-class families sought medical services in hospitals rather than in their own home. This led to increased dissatisfaction with the quality of handy-women nurses and with the education and control of nurses.

Nursing sisterhoods and Christian ladies

Florence Nightingale and other heroines of nursing's history sought to improve the standards of nursing through placing nursing and nurses under the control of religiously motivated, upper-class women of independent means and independent minds. A range of 'sisterhoods' (Abel-Smith 1960, Dingwall *et al.* 1988) developed in the 1840s, supplying home nursing care that emphasised the spiritual and moral concerns of the sick. In London, St John's House Training Institution for Nurses, founded in 1848, took over for a period the organisation of nursing for King's College Hospital, and sisterhood nurses (from the Sisterhood of the Holy Cross, the Protestant Sisters of Charity and the Sisterhood of Mercy of

Devonport and Plymouth) were involved in supplying female nurses to troops in the Crimean war. The pattern of nursing organisation adopted by the sisterhoods became a common model throughout hospitals. Nurses in charge, or sisters, held a supervisory position over nurses and probationary nurses, as well as over ward maids. Ward staff, under the supervision of the sister, carried out domestic as well as medical duties, watching over patients by day and wards by night. Similarly, when working in the community, the nurses and probationers were expected to assist with domestic tasks while the supervisory sisters trained the junior nurses and visited the sick and aged, providing spiritual care. Important differences between the nursing sisters and the junior nurses were that the sisters paid for their own board and lodging and did not receive payment, while the ordinary nurses received payment for their labour. The sisters were deemed to have the responsibility for patients' spiritual welfare. 'An ordinary nurse rarely had the time to consider her patient's spiritual welfare; moreover she was not to be credited with the capacity to steer them towards salvation' (Summers 1988: 60). Thus nursing became a *vocation* for middle-class women and a *job* for women of the working class.

In the 'history as progress' version of nursing's development, it is the philanthropy and reforming zeal of Florence Nightingale, who led a party of female nurses to the Crimean war, and the leaders of the sisterhoods, who introduced a system of organising and training nurses, that ensured nursing's credibility and respectability. Such credibility and respectability was seen as being dependent on the type of woman recruited into the profession. Nurse leaders who did not 'fit' the image of a higher class of women were ignored in nursing's history, as Mary Seacole's treatment exemplifies.

Maggs (1980) has identified the idealised picture of the nurse recruit in the late nineteenth century. Her preferred age was 25–35, mature enough to face the distressing nature of the work yet young enough to be adaptable and fit enough to cope with the physical labour. The probationer was to be 'a Christian lady' willing to undergo a training that was described by one probationer as embracing

> habits of order cleanliness, gentleness and quietness: without these, the theoretical training would be worth nothing, and no true woman would

object to scouring, provided it was for the good of the patient... no woman of refinement of any feeling would deem it degrading.

(Brockbank 1970, cited in Maggs 1980: 21)

Those entering nursing would ideally enter experienced in the domestic and practical arts of cooking, needlework and household management, but unsullied by employment in an industrial context. As Maggs notes, 'such imagery undoubtedly impinged on the ideas held by other groups (doctors, patients) concerning nurses and nursing. It was certainly in the mind of the matron as she set about interviewing prospective trainees' (Maggs 1980: 21). This idealised prescriptive model of the new nurse in the late nineteenth century did not match the reality of the diversity of women who entered nursing, but it is nevertheless an image of considerable power and persistence.

It is not possible here to review the complexity of nursing's history nor the varied histories that can be found. It is important to note, however, that whereas leaders of the sisterhoods and some lady reformers, such as Mary Stanley, fully endorsed the priority given to Godliness in nursing care, albeit based on what Summers (1989) describes as 'a very determined confusion of the notions of social and spiritual superiority' (p. 60), Florence Nightingale did not necessarily share this view. To see Nightingale's interest in nursing reform as solely lady bountiful philanthropy would be to denigrate the robustness of her vocational instruction. Writing on infection, for example, she ridiculed the practice of avoiding contact with patients with infections, noting that 'true nursing ignores infection, except to prevent it. Cleanliness and fresh air from open windows, with unremitting attention to the patient are the only defence a true nurse either asks or needs' (Nightingale 1970 [1859]: 20). Nursing, for Nightingale, was a practical activity as well as a vocation. Her *Notes on Nursing* were written as hints for every woman, since 'every woman is a nurse' (Nightingale 1970 [1859]: 3).

Female nurses in the Crimean War

Nightingale is remembered as a leader of nursing because of the success of the female nurses in the Crimean War. This success was achieved despite conflict between what Summers (1989) has described as two different models of the relationship between working-class women and their employers, one based on the domestic economy of servants living within a household under the patronage and control of the mistress of the house, the other based on the market control of paid labour. It is interesting to note how women's role in a bourgeois morality project may conflict with their role as cheap, replaceable labour, indispensable to capitalism. The conflict between these two models of class relationship posed a problem for relationships between the ladies recruited to lead the Crimean nurses and the paid nurses expected to work under their supervision. According to Summers (1988), Florence Nightingale, in recruiting the first party to the Crimea, sought to reduce the conflict by engaging no 'lady volunteers', recruiting nurses from sisterhoods and hospitals, thus ensuring that all had experience of nursing work.

However, nurses for the second expedition, recruited by Mary Stanley, included more ladies to take supervisory roles. Although the Secretary of State at War, Sidney Herbert, had instructed the second party of nurses that 'no one was to consider herself as in any way above her companions' (cited in Summers 1989: 57), this view was not welcomed by the ladies, who succeeded in effecting control over the paid nurses through recreating the discipline of the Victorian household. Paid nurses were required to act as servants to the ladies. The ladies distanced themselves from the nursing recruits by not wearing their nursing uniforms, being unable to accept a style of dress signifying domestic service for themselves. 'The nurses were not allowed in the wards except under the ladies' supervision' (Summers 1989: 68). This was justified by the needs of the patients. Nurses were trusted neither to carry out medical orders unsupervised nor to resist the intrusion and biasing effect of personal relationships with patients. Familiarity with patients was discouraged and opportunities for personal communication limited. Even meal times and social activities were supervised by the ladies. Those who could not and would not tolerate such control were dismissed (Dingwall *et al.* 1988).

The ladies' view of the appropriate supervisory role for higher-class women, based on their moral superiority and authority, eventually gained favour with the authorities financing the nursing schemes. Ladies as volunteer nurses were able to bring status to nursing because of the unpaid nature of their work, turning nursing into a vocation, religiously sustained and impossible to pursue if 'sullied by thoughts of material gain' (Summers 1988, 1989: 73).

Summers (1989) argues that the concept of a lady in nineteenth century England has to be understood alongside the concept of a non-lady. What distinguishes a lady from a non-lady is not the type of work she does (ladies in the Crimea *did* do the laundry and *did* delouse the patients) but the paid or unpaid status of the worker. Summers quotes Jane Shaw Stewart's remark 'the real dignity of a gentlewoman is a very high and unassailable thing, which silently encompasses her from cradle to grave' (1989: 74). Despite the obfuscation involved in this concept, which ascribes a superior morality to women of a higher class who were themselves financially dependent on a father or husband, Summers notes that the ladies' assumed equality with men of their own status gave them the confidence to argue for more humane treatment of the other women whom they saw as their charges. Paradoxically, the cultural acceptance of ladies' financial dependence meant that it could be completely ignored; the ladies, unlike the ordinary nurses, were not vulnerable employees. Among the ladies were 'women of great intelligence, determination and moral independence' (Summers 1989: 74).

Nursing hierarchies in nineteenth century England

Establishing a female hierarchy within nursing became a class project that gained support in the latter half of the nineteenth century through a perceived need to control the working class. Although few matrons and sisters were of independent means, nursing leadership became an occupation for 'distressed gentlewomen', middle-class ladies who needed to earn their own living. One version of nursing's history is that it did indeed become an occupation for middle-class girls, particularly once training schools were established in the major London teaching hospitals. The Nightingale fund, established after the Crimea, was used to establish the Nightingale School at St Thomas' Hospital. Thus, the control over nursing recruits exercised by higher-class ladies in the Crimea was matched by a similar control over recruitment throughout England. The extent to which the class base of nursing did change is, however, unclear. The majority of recruits to the profession were probably working-class women, made respectable by the rigidity of the control to which they were subjected. Respectable working-class women were recruited to exert control over their own class. Although Maggs found that recruitment in provincial hospitals was not restricted to the idealised image of middle-class femininity (recruits being younger and having more prior work experience than the image suggests), selection and retention were strongly influenced by Matron's perception of attributes incompatible with nursing; 'laziness, indolence, bad education, a lack of dedicated application' (Maggs 1980: 37).

Men in nursing in the nineteenth century

The significance of the parties of female nurses sent to the Crimea in 1854 lay in the fact that female nurses were allowed among the soldiers at all. Male orderlies worked in military hospitals under the direction of male ward sergeants. One of the difficulties with this system was that male orderlies could be called back to the front at any time, thus leaving the hospitals with the task of continually replacing their skilled labour. Lady nurses and their parties had, therefore, to work alongside established patterns of male organisation. The higher class of the ladies would have been an important element in their ability to gain any influence over the male workers. It was, indeed, the incongruity of the ladies' position in relation to what they would have regarded as an inferior class of men that encouraged the ladies' resistance to wearing uniforms. The uniforms allowed all classes and both sexes to make unwarranted assumptions about equality, which could lead, for the ladies, to unwelcome familiarity from medical orderlies. Summers (1989), in quoting one such example of familiarity, notes 'the enormity of the offence lay not so much in the orderly's indirect reference to the lady's innards, but in addressing her at all' (p. 67).

In civilian life, male attendants worked under the (often remote) supervision of medical superintendents in institutions established for the care of the mentally ill and 'mentally subnormal'. Among asylum staff, 'nurse' was a term reserved for women. Dingwall *et al.* (1988) report that from the outset asylum work was dominated by working-class men, the nearest equivalent of the 'handywoman' class in general nursing. This resulted partly from the need for physical strength if patients needed to be forcibly restrained. However, the importance of the economic activities of the asylum should not be overlooked. These men had the kind of low-level skills of agriculture and related workshop production which were essential for the supervision of patient labour. The declining demand for workers in the agricultural sector which freed women for employment in general nursing also released men for the staffing of asylums.

(p. 127)

Although the regimes in some asylums were based on therapeutic models of work and of self and moral discipline, in practice staffing levels meant that many asylums adopted regimes of control staffed by disciplinarian male attendants. Towards the end of the nineteenth century, changes in medical methods of treating mental illness, including a greater use of physical therapies and warranting a greater understanding of biological processes, led medical superintendents to introduce nursing hierarchies modelled on general nursing into the asylums. Matron posts in asylums became available to ambitious women who found their opportunities in the general nursing sector blocked by the appointment of young women to senior posts in hospitals. Such career-orientated women from general nursing were resented by male attendants, who saw their own opportunities blocked.

In voluntary hospitals, male medical attendants also assisted the doctors, mainly with specific activities or as medical students or juniors. Apothecaries were early medical attendants who expanded the scope of their work from mixing and supplying medications to diagnosis and treatment, uniting with physicians and surgeons under the Medical Act 1858 and thus gaining the status of medical men. Although women nurses were recruited partly to carry out the duties released by the change in status of the apothecaries, nurses' work became in practice mainly that of a domestic nature, while apprentice physicians, surgeons or apothecaries assisted with technical procedures and with the observation of patients, activities that were to become the responsibility of nurses in the twentieth century (Dingwall *et al.* 1988).

Male doctors and female nurses in the nineteenth century

The working-class men who staffed the asylums were not the only males to resent the middle-class women – 'daughters of military officers, clergymen, lawyers, and many other connected with the liberal professions; governesses, pupil-teachers, farmers' daughters', whom Dr Greene, the medical superintendent of Berry Wood Asylum, Northampton, claimed to have engaged (cited in Carpenter 1980: 136). Doctors in the London hospitals did not necessarily welcome independently minded senior nurses of their own social class. Although medical developments became increasingly dependent on appropriately trained nurses, the expectations of these women were clearly restricted. Moore (1988: 43) quotes a leading article from *The Times* in 1876, which gives a character sketch of the sort of women seen as suitable for nurse training:

> They are sympathetic and gentle; they have no excessive flow of spirits or range of ideas; they can speak when spoken to, and hold their tongues when it is fit to be silent. They can attend to small matters and bear them in mind. They can take pleasure in small arrangements, so as they have a use or priority. They can attach significance to such superficial matters as dirt or smell. They can believe there is something in orders which they cannot themselves understand. They can mediate between the doctor and the patient, being a faithful assistant to the former and a kind, but not oppressive, friend and advisor to the latter.
>
> (Moore 1988: 43)

This brief account of nursing before 1900 can, as already indicated, be interpreted in different ways. The 'history as progress' view of nursing sees the attraction of higher-class women of sensibility into leadership positions in nursing as a means of ensuring that nursing became a profession for the respectable good woman. Such respectability was guaranteed through a hierarchical system of management and education developed through the efforts of individuals, particularly Florence Nightingale, and made possible through the dedicated work of lady volunteers during the Crimean war.

Sociological approaches to nursing history: feminist accounts

Feminist accounts of nursing's history, while deploring the ladies' use of claims to spiritual superiority to support their social superiority (a superiority dependent on patriarchal social structures), would identify the importance of the development of nursing as a respectable profession for women in securing economic independence for middle-class women. Upper-class philanthropy, seeking to reform nursing, led, it could be argued, to an avenue for independently minded women to seek employment outside the domestic sphere. However, dominant constructions of women as feeble-minded and subservient, favoured by many doctors, severely restricted the opportunities available for women as nurses to exercise independent judgement. Thus, women working as subservient nurses reinforced the patriarchal nature of the 'knowledge project', whereby it is men who are regarded as the rational creators of knowledge about the world. Women's exclusion from science and confinement to the domestic sphere was maintained even within the hospital. For some women, therefore, a greater challenge than nursing was to seek qualification as a doctor. Florence Nightingale, however, expressed the view that medicine and nursing were two separate spheres of activity, which could appropriately be divided between the sexes. Such a view was a feature of Victorian culture; the ideology was that men were breadwinners, active in the public sphere, while women remained in the private sphere, occupied with the responsibilities of home making (Hannam 1997).

Nursing and the labour market

An analysis of occupational change based on approaches that emphasise the importance of the economy in societal change would identify several economic factors. The declining need for agricultural labour released both men and women into the labour market. Men and women accustomed to traditional agricultural hierarchies, like those accustomed to domestic service, were seen as particularly suitable for the 'hospital as household' model of health care adopted both in the asylums, the principal place of employment for men, and in the hospitals. Despite the expressed intention of many hospitals to recruit middle-class Christian ladies of mature years, unsullied by employment beyond the domestic sphere or charitable works, the reality was probably that most recruits, at least in the provinces, were young women from the respectable working class (Maggs 1980). Male asylum attendants were from a similar background, although some accounts present a less positive view, describing asylum recruits as unemployable elsewhere (Carpenter 1980).

Class analyses would note the importance of the role of women and of the respectable working class in controlling the sick. The higher class of the lady volunteers in the Crimea ensured that women could work as equals, if not as superiors, among male orderlies, a strategy similarly adopted later in the mental asylums, where women's appointments to senior positions served to control men of an inferior class and to restrict the wage levels. Female labour could be considerably cheaper than male.

There is as yet no adequate history of nursing that explores what nurses actually did during the nineteenth century, either before or after the process of reform. Abel-Smith's (1960) major historical work specifically notes the nature of nurses' work as an omission. The activities of female nurses, particularly female nurses recruited for their respectability, must have been constrained by gender expectations of the time, particularly expectations associated with sexuality. It is clear that the ratio of nurses to patients in the Crimea made the provision of intimate physical care almost impossible, but it is probable that middle-class women would have found it exceedingly difficult to care physically for young men's bodies. Both at war and in the asylums, physical care for the men would probably have been provided by the male attendants. It was the domestic labour of nursing that made the work women's work, despite the fact that the reduction in such domestic labour for trained nurses was, for Florence Nightingale, an explicit aim. In the Crimea, nurses certainly found opportunities to offer spiritual care, practised mainly through providing comfort for the dying.

Thus, choosing to nurse in the late nineteenth century may have been a relatively common activity among a wide range of young women, albeit for different reasons. Choosing to nurse would have depended on what options there were available for women at that time. Apart from domestic service in their own or in another's household, there were few. Nursing offered opportunities to women of all classes. For higher-class women, nursing offered, with the implicit support of government, considerable power over their own sex. Within nursing, particularly in the voluntary hospitals, higher-class women established work patterns imbued with symbols and rituals of morality to maintain superiority over other women.

Men, however, would not have chosen to *nurse* since this was a title restricted mainly to women. Male attendants may have performed similar work, but without the public associations with moral respectability and discipline so important to their female counterparts. Despite the stress on the links between nursing and feminine attributes, links that were successfully used to confirm dominant Victorian constructions of femininity, asylum work does not appear to have been viewed as contrary to the accepted notions of masculinity. Indeed, the physical nature of the work and the accepted hierarchical pattern of the working-class male deferring to the authority of men from a higher social status (in this instance, medical men) suggest that male 'nurses' in the nineteenth century conformed to accepted patterns of masculinity within male hierarchies grounded in economic differences. Women's emphasis on distinctions between women in terms of morality and respectability may result from the insubstantial nature of women's economic power. Women in the nineteenth century were not economically independent; lacking direct economic control, the ladies had to maintain class superiority through control over the morality project. Nursing became the symbol of women's superiority and moral control.

Nursing in the twentieth century: 1900–45

Many significant events including female suffrage, nurse registration, increasing medicalisation and two world wars influenced both the development of nursing and the development of opportunities for women in the first half of the twentieth century. This part of the chapter focuses on the influence of changes in health care, the influence of war, the nurse registration movement, and the effect on men in nursing.

Changes in health care

Features of the Victorian era that continued well into the twentieth century included the importance of the voluntary hospitals with their now established 'Nightingale' system of independent control of nursing by a nursing hierarchy headed by matron. Although Nightingale (1970 [1859]) herself certainly emphasised the importance of far more than character in her own *Notes on Nursing*, the enactment of her principles of nursing management led to the system in which dedicated single women were trained in the appropriate personal qualities for nursing. The dedication demanded by their vocation meant that, until World War Two, voluntary hospital nurses were normally required to leave on marriage.

Poor Law hospitals, administered through public assistance committees, were responsible for elderly people and those chronically ill. Here the 'handy-woman' class of nurses supervised the sick and the untrained nurses. After the 1929 Local Government Act, most Poor Law hospitals became the responsibility of local authorities, with some municipal hospitals serving a public health function, protecting the public from the spread of transmittable diseases such as tuberculosis. In many of these hospitals, as well as in the psychiatric sector, nurses, although relatively unaffected by the nursing reforms that brought status to nurses in the voluntary hospitals, 'exercised considerable "front-line" power independent of doctors and administrators' (Bellaby and Oribabor 1980: 166).

The increasing medicalisation of health care, however, began to alter patterns of hospital work from the early twentieth century. Developments in medical knowledge brought an increase in medical specialisation and an increase in the need for specialised skills, including skills in using new equipment to produce diagnostic information (X-rays, for example) and skills in administering new forms of therapy. Although some new professions, including physiotherapy and radiography, developed, techniques hitherto carried out by doctors and medical students (taking blood pressures, monitoring intravenous infusions and dressing wounds) became part of the work of the nurse. Nursing tasks such as the maintenance of ward hygiene increasingly became the responsibility of domestic staff, and nursing duties became increasingly controlled by medical practitioners. Bellaby and Oribabor argue that as the technical subordination of nursing developed, so the nursing structure pioneered by the reformers in the larger voluntary hospitals was eroded from within... the structure of domination was changing. In the 'old' pattern, a nurse acted on the orders of the ward sister or matron, even if to service the orders of a doctor: she remained part of a corps in her daily interaction with medicine. In the 'emergent' pattern, she was a technical assistant in one of several different teams each commanded by medicine, usually by a single consultant.

(1980: 164)

Matron appeared to be losing control of her charges to the decision making power of individual men. The 'incipient erosion of the inner discipline of the nursing corps helps explain the tenacity with which matrons and national leaders in the 1930s defended matron's control of training, hours of work and even leisure' (Bellaby and Oribabor 1980: 164). The medicalisation of nursing tasks had extensive consequences. It challenged the matron's status, challenged the adequacy of the education system that stressed the importance of character rather than knowledge or skills, and challenged the unity of nursing through necessitating an increase in the number of untrained assistants (eventually leading to the recognition of a need for a 'lower grade' of nurse) and through requiring individual nurses to work under the variable instructions of individual consultants. The movement towards two grades of nurse was resisted by matrons seeking to retain a united corps, often through retaining 'basic' and domestic tasks as work for the learner nurses, whose own education they were prepared to neglect in favour of retaining nursing control over the work.

Furthermore, the increased effectiveness of medical interventions led to a widening class base among hospitalised patients. The established pattern of nursing hierarchy and nurse training ensured a compliant workforce taught to encourage equivalent humility and passivity among the predominantly lower-class patients. Nurses trained in obedience and respectability in order to instil similar virtues in their patients found themselves in ambiguous relationships with middle-class patients who took their own respectability for granted and expected to be obeyed rather than to obey. Senior nurses did not want their ward nurses treated as servants by the patients in their care. As the influence of sisterhoods within the hospitals decreased, however, any spiritual or moral basis for control over both nurses and patients became less relevant.

Matrons and sisters could no longer rely on occupying a dominant class position among their patients, and nursing could be seen as losing its control over the 'morality project'.

The effects of war: nurses, VADs and health visitors

In the early twentieth century, in the hospital sector, it was the relationship between higher-class women and nurses that challenged the adequacy of 'a good nurse is a good woman' as a model for nursing as a professional activity or even as an occupation. During World War One, additional nursing labour was provided mainly by women of the Voluntary Aid Detachments (VADs) who worked in military and auxiliary hospitals under contract to the War Office. As Dingwall *et al.* note:

> The VADs tended to come from upper- and middle-class backgrounds, partly because many of them were unpaid... They posed a considerable threat to the established order of nursing, especially because the patients rarely distinguished between them and the trained nurses. The lady nurses saw the possibility of their exclusive position being diluted while the ordinary nurses saw themselves as likely to be further downgraded by this influx of women from more privileged backgrounds.

> (1988: 73)

Vera Brittain (1978) records her resentment of the defensive and restrictive way in which she was treated by nurses in civilian hospitals (in contrast to the responsibilities she was delegated in military hospitals), attributing her treatment to a fear of VADs becoming too knowledgeable and a mistaken view that vast numbers of experienced VADs would wish to continue in nursing in peacetime, thus threatening the status of those already in the profession. Brittain saw such fears as groundless, commenting that

> all but a very few VADs were only too thankful when the War was over to quit a singularly backward profession for their own occupations and interests, but many 'trained women' having no such interests themselves could not believe that others were attracted to them.

> (1978: 309)

The strengths of the nursing reforms of the Nightingale era, which introduced a powerful system of nursing management and training, came to be seen as repressive and restrictive by the class of women responsible for the nineteenth century nursing reforms.

Some higher-class women, however, retained an interest in health care through a public health role as health visitors. State sponsorship of health visiting as an occupation grew through concerns for the welfare of children after the poor health of young working-class males was identified through army recruitment for the Boer War and World War One. Although health visiting originated in sanitary reform, health visitors became more involved in maternity and child welfare services after 1914. Health visiting was part of a movement to improve the health of the population through environmental health measures and through what has been characterised in sociology as the surveillance of working-class homes and families by middle-class women (Bloor and McIntosh 1990). Health visitor training schemes were available for those with a medical or nursing background and for those without. It was not until 1963 that the Council for Training of Health Visitors decided that only registered general nurses were eligible for health visiting training, limiting opportunities for non-nurses and for nurses in psychiatry or other specialisms. Throughout the century, health visitors and nurses were educated differently. White identified two important differences. Health visitors were

> educated in social health and social policy, building upon scientific principles. In contrast to this, other nurses were trained in curative medicine by didactic methods which concentrated on procedures rather than principles.

> (1985: 162)

Not all health visitors, however, would have seen themselves as nurses, and not all nurses would have seen health visiting as part of nursing. The delimiting of 'nurse' and 'non-nurse' became particularly important through nursing's pursuit of professionalism through registration.

The registration movement

The struggle for a state licensing system for nurses, ensuring that the occupation would be closed to anyone lacking an identified set of credentials, began in the 1880s but gained considerable attention during World War One, partly as a result of concerns about the activities of the VADs. A state-supported, legally binding form of credentialism is seen as an important characteristic of a profession (Porter 1998, Wilkinson and Miers 1999). Witz (1992) has studied the registration campaign, drawing on Weberian analyses of professionalisation as occupational closure. She uses registration as a 'professionalising project' to identify the way in which gender provided a source of solidarity and collective action for women involved in professionalising projects. Nursing registration as a professionalising project did not, however, promote solidarity among nurses. The leading protagonist for registration, Mrs Bedford-Fenwick, argued for the autonomy for nurses over their own education and their own sphere of work, that is, autonomy from the control of medical practitioners. Mrs Bedford-Fenwick was an ardent supporter of women's rights, and she sought to free nursing from (male) medical control through seeking to ensure that the control of the education of nursing was placed in a state-legitimated body, controlled by nurses, but 'external to and independent of the existing internal systems of control located within the institutional framework of the hospital' (Witz 1992: 147). Unsurprisingly, those nurses who benefitted most from the existing system of control within hospitals, namely the matrons (supported by Florence Nightingale), were against registration.

Dingwall et al. (1988: 79) have argued that Mrs Bedford-Fenwick was really interested in reorganising private, home nursing along the lines of the organisation of the medical profession. Registration could give women an independent and autonomous status as nurses, free to work for a range of employers in a range of settings. Nursing, as an independent profession, could thus become an attractive high status occupation able to attract middle-class recruits, without the restrictions imposed through a hierarchical management system dependent on the employment needs of particular hospitals.

It was not until the nursing hierarchy within the voluntary hospitals saw their own status being threatened by a possible influx of middle-class women VADs after the war that the matrons' opposition to registration declined. A Nurse Registration Bill was eventually passed in 1919, and at the same time a bill was passed establishing a College of Nursing. These two bills were supported by different sides of the registration debate. The College of Nursing was established as a means of co-operation between hospitals with training schools, thus ensuring that the voluntary hospital élite maintained a collective professional arena in which they were able to maintain control. The Registration Act should have given nursing, as a profession, autonomy above these élite hospitals, but although the maintenance of a register of nursing became a state responsibility, there was no power granted to make 'Registered Nurse' a precondition of employment. The unity of nursing was diluted through the creation of supplementary sections of the Register (male nurses, mental nurses, sick children's nurses and fever nurses).

Dingwall *et al.* (1988) and Witz (1992) share the view that state registration represented a failure for pro-registrationist nurses. Witz (1992) saw registration as a dual closure strategy that failed. Registration did not restrict nursing to an élite group of highly educated professionals – untrained labour continuing to work alongside nurses – and registration did not give nurses autonomy from doctors and the freedom to define their own boundaries. Nurses did gain a majority of representatives (16 out of 25) on the central statutory body, the General Nursing Council (GNC), but it became a body with few powers as the rules it devised had to receive ministerial approval. The GNC gained powers to regulate the conduct of examinations but not their content, and the Council had no powers over pay and employment conditions.

It is worth exploring some of the subtleties of gendered assumptions that lay behind the arguments about registration. Mrs Bedford-Fenwick's vision of 'a rigorous training modelled on that of the medical profession, with its pattern of a general foundation followed by specialisation and indifferent to the staffing needs of particular institutions' (Dingwall *et al.* 1988: 90) is a vision that is still debated. Criticisms of the vision on the grounds that it disregarded the labour needs of the Poor Law hospitals and the asylums and that it served the interests of the middle class, who could afford such education, may also sound familiar.

Some of the medical profession's arguments against registration, however, will not sound acceptable today. Dingwall *et al.*

(1988) quote a range of views from the 1904 Select Committee on the Registration of Nurses. Dr Norman Moore from St Bartholomew's Hospital thought book learning was of little value to a nurse. The Victorian 'separate spheres' theory of the complementarity of men's and women's qualities led to the view that a doctor would be engaged for his skill, a nurse for her virtue (House of Commons 1904). The registrationist vision of an autonomous nursing profession was a challenge 'not merely to the particular relations between doctors and nurses but to the whole theoretical foundations of the gender order in health care' (Dingwall *et al.* 1988: 83). However, nursing had already established itself as an activity that confirmed rather than challenged the gender order in health care and beyond. Nightingale accepted the complementarity of the gender order, although she did not agree that physiological knowledge, for example, was the preserve of medical men (Nightingale 1970 [1859]).

Mrs Bedford-Fenwick's view of the potential for women's and nursing's autonomy challenged the accepted binary and relational view of gender in that her view suggested that women could not only be knowledgeable and skilled, but also equal to and not dependent upon men. In the twentieth century, however, women seeking challenges to the gender order found varied opportunities in employment and education. In health care, their options extended to medicine and the growing range of allied professions. Nursing ceased to be the obvious choice.

Men in nursing 1900–45

The fact that men in nursing also presented a challenge to the gendered order in health care is something that is widely overlooked. The challenge was easily ignored by simply failing to acknowledge men as nurses. Men had to be registered as general nurses on a supplementary part of the register after the Nurse Registration Act. Milligan (1993) reports that no men registered as general nurses until 1922, and only two general hospitals were approved to train male nurses by 1924 (Greene 1992/3). The challenge that men in nursing presented in the early twentieth century was their self-perception as workers and employees, untroubled by ideas of vocation or profession. Male attendants in mental asylums followed male workers in the industrial sector and used unions to protect their interests, adopting an industrial rather than a domestic view of organisation. Medical superintendents had sponsored the development of an Association of Workers in Asylums in 1897, and this organisation supported the Asylum Officers Superannuation Act 1909, which was an attempt to improve the attendants' conditions of work by requiring employers to introduce pension schemes. Many schemes were, however, introduced on a contributory basis, which were seen as effecting a wage cut. Since general nurses in the public hospital sector had better conditions of service, this prompted male attendants to form a new National Asylum Workers Union, which affiliated to the Labour Party in 1914 and to the TUC in 1923 (Dingwall *et al.* 1988: 130).

Gender divisions within the asylum workforce (and the growing sector for the care of the mentally deficient, separated from mental illness provision following the Mental Deficiency Act in 1913) increased through an increasing emphasis on medical treatment including surgery, insulin therapy and electrical treatments. These therapies required some knowledge of general nursing techniques, which led to an increased influence of general nursing models of management and to an emphasis on the importance of a double qualification for those who sought senior positions. Although, in the first instance, female general nurses may have gained senior positions in mental health asylums, the double qualification requirement encouraged men to train as general nurses, eventually facilitating male nurses' mobility as managers.

Although mental nurses welcomed registration, the Medico-Psychological Association (MPA) already had its own certificate for mental nurses, which was accepted by the GNC for entry onto the supplementary register. The GNC did not accept the MPA certificate as the route to registration, however, and introduced its own certificate, the two qualifications competing for some time. Although the creation of the GNC may have alleviated staffing difficulties for a short time in the 1920s, through facilitating female nurses' movement into mental health services, the services suffered through lack of public funds in the 1930s. Wages and conditions deteriorated, and employers sought further supplies of cheap labour, for example from Ireland. Despite changes in the rhetoric of psychiatric care, emphasising more holistic care, staff in mental and mental deficiency hospitals were poorly educated and given little status within the nursing profession. Indeed, the General Nursing Council opposed the incorporation of mental deficiency nursing in 1919. Unsurprisingly, therefore, male nurses in these neglected areas adopted little of the rhetoric of nursing's claims, as vocation or profession. Male nurses were workers and custodians in settings largely free from the daily surveillance of higher-class men or women, as either colleagues, superiors or clients. The strengths and weakness of male nurses developing their own ways of working have yet to be explored.

Summary

Some trends can be identified from this overview of a century of nursing. Whereas in the nineteenth century a higher class of women led the reform of nursing so that it could be a profession of choice for middle-class women, in the twentieth century nursing progressively lost the support of upper- and middle-class women, who sought greater freedom through education and widening employment opportunities. As service sector and clerical jobs increased for women, choice was increasing for all classes of woman. Attempts to improve the status of nursing through professional credentialism did not result in educational gains and autonomy from the medical profession. Instead, the importance of meeting the labour needs of local hospitals reinforced the controlling general nursing hierarchy in each hospital. Isolated in hospitals, nursing leadership became increasingly narrow and increasingly defensive of its work-based education system posited on obedience and procedures rather than principles. Support for the repetition of tasks as a method of developing skills and for the practical nature of nursing as an activity led to the rejection and denigration of nursing by women with wider interests.

If nursing was losing status in the twentieth century, however, it was not in the eyes of the public. Nursing participated in a class-based Victorian morality project with considerable success and in so doing became closely aligned with the ministering angel imagery and the mythology of matron. The public power of such mythology, and the fact that women and nurses continue to tend the sick as they always have done, gives nursing a permanently valued and devalued place in British culture. It is a place shared by women, women as mothers, women as handy-women, good women. In a society in which secular processes such as labour market relations, political representation and legislation became the means for ensuring fairness and enforcing morality, ladies who improved the status of nursing through their role in the nineteenth century morality project became just ladies, neither bountiful nor even educated. The twentieth century widened educational and employment opportunities for women. Nurses became increasingly the handmaidens of medical men. In attempting to preserve a hitherto successful method of hospital management, a dominant group of nurses sought to exclude others (men, VADs and mental deficiency attendants) as non-nurses.

If nursing ceases to be an attractive occupation for women, its status as a role for good women becomes threatened. Nurses' sense of their own value is reduced. The diversity in femininities hidden in nursing's history can be located in different views on gender and the knowledge project. Despite Mrs Bedford-Fenwick's advocacy of educational reform and despite Florence Nightingale's clear recognition of the importance of nurses' understanding of laws of hygiene, nursing came to define itself as a practical art, grounded in women's practical skills. It was in the doctor's interests to ensure that nurses developed practical rather than cognitive skills. Such a view conformed to the dominant expectations of both men and women. As higher educational (academic) qualifications became a valuable form of social mobility and social status for women as well as men, nursing's apparent isolation from academic concerns allowed educated women to distance themselves from nursing and from its particular forms of anti-intellectual, repressive femininity. Nurses were excluded, and excluded themselves, from the knowledge project.

Male nurses were probably, for the first half of the twentieth century, considerably disadvantaged by the dominance of women and by models of general nursing. Nevertheless, although little is known about patterns of male nurse recruitment and employment before the NHS, men's exclusion from, and indifference to, the intricacies of hospital general nursing traditions may well have ensured that they were well placed to take advantage of post-war conditions and developments in nursing. As Chapter 8 illustrates, nursing's hierarchical system of control over its own recruits inhibited nurses' ability to develop as leaders and managers in changing systems of health care.

5 Nursing in the NHS

Introduction

This chapter continues to explore the relationship between constructions of femininity and masculinity, and recruitment to nursing, concentrating on the latter half of the twentieth century. The demand for nurses to staff the British National Health Service (NHS) after World War Two coincided with two conflicting trends affecting women. On the one hand, after the disruption of war, women returned home to be mothers. On the other, women's participation in education and employment increased. This chapter focuses on the effects on nursing of changes in women's role and on women's increasing educational opportunities, as well as on the changing role of men in nursing.

Women's changing role

Some constructions of femininity examined in Chapters 1 and 2 are missing from the images of nursing and of gender presented in Chapter 4. Where, for example, is the sexy nurse? Such an image was relatively hidden under nursing's images of nineteenth century respectability. The overtly sexualising and romanticising of nursing through media images of hyperfemininity developed comparatively recently. The *Carry On* films and the 1950s and 60s' television series *Emergency Ward 10* (1957–67) and *Dr Kildare* popularised images of nursing (Kalisch and Kalisch 1982a, 1982b).

Hallam (1998) suggests that, at this time, the public image of nursing functioned as a discourse of femininity. In the post-war era, public images of nursing drew on conventional codes of femininity that resulted in the renegotiation of nursing's 'ethos of public service as feminine service to medicine' (p. 41). 'Sexy nurse' imagery appeared at the same time as both a post-war emphasis on the importance of women's role as mothers and an increase in the proportion of women taking employment outside the home. Class and status divisions between women acquired new cultural manifestations as women's educational opportunities increased and their work and domestic roles changed. Hallam (1998) notes that the social diversity of women entering nursing increased, but higher-class women seeking professional roles and higher education sought opportunities outside nursing. Hence, before considering the effects of social change on nursing, it would be helpful to explore the changes in women's roles and opportunities that occurred in the decades following World War Two. I have found a contemporary sociology text, *Women's Two Roles*, written by two American sociologists, Alva Myrdal and Viola Klein, which was first published in 1956 and minimally revised in 1968, particularly helpful in the following analysis.

Myrdal and Klein (1968) identified two major changes in the position of women in developed Western democracies during the twentieth century, the first being the increasing admission of women into 'masculine' jobs, and the second the 'endeavour of a growing number of women to combine family and employment'. Whereas in the nineteenth century, it was only upper- and middle-class women who were not employed outside the home, in the twentieth century, as the wages of the working man rose,

> many working-class women left the labour market, since it was felt to be an important element in a higher standard of living that wives and mothers should be able to stay at home, like the women in more privileged social groups. It eventually fell to the women in the urban middle class to symbolise the more systematic return to economic productivity, by entering paid employment.
>
> (Myrdal and Klein 1968: 1–2)

The perceived importance of women staying at home derived from more than just a concern to demonstrate the affluence of the family. There were concerns for the effects of mothers' employment on the health and wellbeing of children and raised expectations concerning the importance and demands of the skills of housewifery. Two images featured strongly in advertisements in women's magazines in the 1950s and 60s: 'the lady of leisure', a feminine ideal deriving from the privileges of the aristocracy, and the hard-working housewife, an image that demonstrated a woman's commitment to her family. By the 1950s, however, an additional form of femininity was developing among middle-class women, that of the 'woman with a career'. It sat uncomfortably alongside the other two ideal feminine roles, both of which continued to thrive. Individual women, depending on their social position, struggled in different ways with the advantages, disadvantages and unreality of all three of these idealised femininities – hard-working housewife, lady of leisure and woman with a career.

'Career woman' became a growing phenomenon of the second half of the twentieth century, bringing with her public debate focused on the role of mothers in the workforce. In the 1950s, it was widely assumed that finding emotional fulfillment in marriage was central to women's happiness. Hence the appropriate stage in family life for women to return to work was debated through a concern for women's welfare as well as for the welfare of children. Uncertainty about their role promoted divisions and diversity among women. Myrdal and Klein note that in the middle period of the twentieth century, at a time of partial emancipation of women,

> much of women's envy of men, which undoubtedly was a strong undercurrent in the earlier feminist movement, has changed its direction and turned into envy of one group of women against another: working women begrudge housewives their freedom to do things in their own time and in their own way... whereas housewives envy employed women their financial independence, the great variety of their social contacts, and their sense of purpose.
>
> (1968: 10)

For young women in the 1940s and 50s, employment before marriage became the norm. Young women led public lives in the company of men before retiring from the labour market in order to start a family. Both men and women in the new service industries could find the workplace an important source of romantic possibilities. In Britain, it was the wartime experience that confirmed that mothers were both able and willing to work outside the home. 'Nine hundred thousand women with domestic ties did part-time work and 1,000,000 women not counted in the above total were engaged in unpaid voluntary war work' (Myrdal and Klein 1968: 52). Immediately post-war, however, married women returned to work in the home. Only 18 per cent of married women living with their husbands were in paid work; women had left their jobs partly to release the work for the men returning from the armed forces, partly because the wartime nurseries closed and partly to raise more children. Nevertheless, after an initial post-war decline, the number of married women in employment rose rapidly. The total number of women in employment rose from 6,620,000 in 1947 to 7,650,000 in 1957 and 8,400,000 in 1965, married women seeking employment accounting for most of the increase. 'While married women were 41 per cent of the female labour force in 1950, they were 54 per cent in 1965' (Myrdal and Klein 1968: 54). Census data for 1961 show that 35 per cent of all practising nurses were married, which Myrdal and Klein see as a 'major breakthrough in a profession formerly confined to spinsters' (p. 58).

Nursing and women's changing work experiences

At the inception of the NHS, most nurses, apart from those in services for the mentally ill and mentally handicapped, were young single women who worked full time, and most senior nurses were spinsters who had continuous service as nurses. The Briggs Report notes a considerable change over the post-war decades until, by 1971, there were 126,486 part-time staff in the hospital service compared with 65,833 in 1963 (Briggs 1972: 119). A survey conducted to inform the Briggs Committee showed that, in 1971,

> In keeping with trends in the female labour force generally, more and more female nurses and midwives break their career at the birth of their first child, return when circumstances allow, often on a part-time basis in the first instance, and gradually increase the contribution they make to the profession as their children grow older.
>
> (p. 121)

It was the increased participation rate of older, married women and the increased use of part-time labour that helped to overcome the shortage of nurses at the time of the development of the NHS. An increase in male recruitment and the recruitment of student and pupil nurses from the Commonwealth and Ireland also reduced the labour shortage.

Despite this upsurge in employment, the consequences for women, both in nursing and elsewhere, were not all positive. Childcare was still considered a mother's job. The NHS has been particularly slow to become a supportive employee of women with children, despite its dependence on women workers. White collar employment burgeoned, but female clerical and secretarial workers took subordinate roles in male-dominated hierarchies, a pattern that appeared to be replicated in health care. Hallam (1998) notes that post-war nursing recruitment literature emphasised 'the hospital as a setting for fun and romance, played out against a backdrop of life and death struggle, echoing the narrative strategies of television melodramas and doctor/nurse romances', (p. 38). Myrdal and Klein cite work by Parrish (1962), based on American data, suggesting that there was a post-war decline in the number of women in the most prestigious professions, attributed to a shift in women's preferences.

> High level intellectual activity has suffered under the impact of earlier marriage, a rising rate of marriage and earlier family formation. The ever-increasing participation of women in the labour force is achieved, it seems, through their willingness to accept low and medium-skilled occupations – either short-term or long-term – in preference to more ambitious career plans which might in the long run conflict with the family role.
>
> (Myrdal and Klein 1968: 66)

Professional women with children who did choose to pursue their career alongside family responsibilities during the 1950s and 60s would not necessarily have received support from other women. Myrdal and Klein note a view of the 1950s and 60s that 'to some extent, to this day a married woman who has a career other than that of housewife is "fallen from grace" and deserving of sympathy' (p. 89). Given the exacting expectations of motherhood and society's willingness to blame working mothers for any issue perceived as a social problem, it would not be surprising for women to have had an ambivalent attitude towards work. Women, as adaptable and flexible workers, took part-time and short-term work, which suited both their families and their employers, but married women could thus be seen as uncommitted and disinterested workers, lacking an appropriate sense of responsibility. Nursing was slow to change its self-image of vocationalism, resting on the dedication of single women.

In the 1940s and 50s, the powerful ideologies of male provider responsibilities, middle-class women's role as ladies of leisure and home as a conspicuous consumption status symbol were particularly strong among the families of the young women most likely to continue into higher education and to consider the responsibilities of professional work. For such women, the difficulties of reconciling the expectations of 'career woman', 'mother' and 'wife' were particularly acute. Myrdal and Klein cite a quotation from Komarovsky (1946) as expressing a view felt by many. An American girl student noted, 'My family had expected me to become Madame Curie and Hedy Lamarr wrapped up in one' (Myrdal and Klein 1968: 138). The respondents in Komarovsky's study found that many girl students found it easier to 'play dumb' on dates, not out of a belief in the superiority of men but through acknowledging a convention that masculine illusions are not to be disturbed.

In nursing, masculine illusions were not disturbed. The wartime and post-war demand for nursing labour was met by lowering the entry gate for nursing. In 1939, the minimum education test for entry to nursing was dropped and an open access policy was introduced. Despite continued pressure from the GNC, the Ministry of Health refused to allow the reintroduction of a minimum standard for nursing recruits until 1962. Even then, the minimum standard specified was two GCE O levels or success in a selection test. Minimum entry requirements for entrance into psychiatric nursing were delayed until 1965. Although some hospitals set their own standards at a considerably higher level, the educational standards of those recruited to nursing at the inception of the NHS and for subsequent decades was low. Only 13.6 per cent of general nursing recruits had more than three O levels in 1963/64, a proportion that had risen to 58.1 per cent by 1969/70. In psychiatric and mental handicap nursing, the percentages were 11.4 per cent and 24.5 per cent respectively (Briggs 1972: 59). Although both the GNC and the Royal College of Nursing (RCN) officially supported the reintroduction of a minimum educational standard, many senior nurses, particularly those with responsibility for staffing the service, were ambivalent. The issue of educational standards was complicated by the introduction of a Roll of nurses in 1943, thus formalising two grades, pupil nurses receiving a practical training for entry on the Roll and student nurses receiving a longer training for entry on the Register.

Internal pressures to raise nurses' educational levels were regularly counteracted by those within nursing who adopted a defensive attitude to raising standards, arguing that since *they* were successfully working as nurses without educational qualifications, there was no obvious need for a change. Unfortunately, such arguments demonstrated the isolation of nursing from general educational trends, which were for a continual rise in educational standards, particularly among professionalising workers. Farnworth, in 1952, published the results of a survey on 'The social prestige of nursing', showing that, unsurprisingly, nursing was losing popularity among daughters of the upper and middle classes. Nursing ceased to be a recommended profession for bright girls, who found that their parents and schools emphasised the importance of their intellectual development. While bright girls learnt to value the (masculine) world of ideas, nurses devalued the relevance of theory for their work, which was seen as being rooted in practical skills. White (1985) reports that scepticism within nursing about the place of particularly intelligent girls was widespread, appearing even in prize-winning essays:

> Unfortunately... the really brilliant girls have the wrong temperament for the work. Their alert, quick, intense minds accompany impatient and intolerant natures, and being rather excitable and erratic people they are the types prone to panic.
>
> (Simson 1953: 899)

Creating a feminine intellectual élite

But the really brilliant girls were not choosing nursing. Middleton's (1987) work, using case studies to explore school experiences of girls in the 1950s and 60s, illustrates the ways in which the organisation of schools through 'streaming' influenced girls' perceptions of femininity and appropriate models of womanhood. Within the top streams, girls of predominantly middle-class backgrounds developed 'intellectual' subcultures 'based on a virginal model of female sexuality' and a 'model of intellectuality' based on fantasies about academic/artistic bohemia (Middleton 1987: 79). Although writing about New Zealand women, the processes described were similar to the experiences of

British women. Middleton notes that, for academic girls, 'the process of cultural reproduction was, at least in part, one of acquiring the "know-how" to become the wife of a professional man' (p. 79).

The women in Middleton's study note the contradictions they experienced through dealing with parental, school and peer models of femininity. One woman found that she had to deny her Maori background and culture in order to study the 'top stream' subjects (French and Latin). One way to resist the dominant model of intellectuality presented by the school was to enact 'an exaggerated display of sexuality – assuming the trappings of "tartiness"' (p. 86). For the top stream girls, their model of sexuality comprised 'romantic attachments and fantasies of relationships with artistic, bohemian, intellectual men'. Their choice of school subjects would enable them to become interesting, sensitive and artistic women, or bring them into contact, through higher education, with successful professional men. Their code of sexual morality both protected the girls from becoming pregnant and enabled parents to protect their own ambitions for their daughters. One participant in Middleton's research acknowledged how her father's and her own ambition led her into a professional career:

Obviously if you think you have an intelligent daughter I suppose you don't want her to marry a drainlayer. Part of this thing was that I would go to university, I would have a career on my own which would make me more interesting and all the rest of it. It wasn't so much that I would have a wonderful life myself – that's part of it, but still there was this fact that I would make some brilliant professional man an exciting wife.

(1987: 84)

The model of intellectuality perpetuated through much of British higher education can be seen as being dependent upon a construction of practical skills as separate from and indeed inferior to intellectual activity (in the same way as academic girls constructed their own sexuality in aesthetic terms in contrast to 'others" status as 'tarts'). Hence while 'bright' girls turned away from nursing, which was often seen as a 'soft option' (Doyal 1995: 169), nurses perpetuated their anti-education bias by insisting on a practical training for a practical job. White (1985) reports that, in a survey by Carter in the early 1950s of 65 nurses with degrees, many felt that they had to hide their academic qualifications. Unsurprisingly, attempts to establish degree level education for nurses throughout the 1950s and 60s were slow to succeed, partly through nursing's own reluctance to accept universities' freedom to control their own courses and partly through a general reluctance on the part of the academic world, governments and other professional groups to accept that nursing necessitated degree level preparation. White (1985) reports on the unsuccessful attempts to establish a Nursing Research Council in the 1950s. It proved impossible even to find anyone willing to act as Chair for such a body.

Class, curriculum and caring

Skeggs (1986, 1997) has identified the close links between class, curriculum and caring in her study of young women following caring courses in further education. She argues that, from the 1930s to the 1960s, curricula were designed to meet the perceived needs of different social classes. The working classes were seen as being potentially dangerous and disreputable, and women, particularly mothers, were seen as important in maintaining respectability. Working-class women, therefore, needed training in their caring role. Women of different classes were offered different opportunities to learn different domestic and feminine 'arts' (literature for the A stream girls, cookery for those in the lower forms). The result was a 'mapping of class-based divisions onto practical and academic education' (Skeggs 1997: 49). Both Skeggs and Middleton make use of Bourdieu's concept of 'cultural capital' to show how both educational success and femininities can be used as resources that can be employed to produce real social effects. Bourdieu (1986) sees education as being a vital source of cultural capital.

Nursing's cultural capital is ambiguous, and whether or not nursing would appear to offer men or women a cultural resource depends on the available alternatives. In the post-war years, nursing may have become a soft and unattractive option to bright middle-class girls, but it still had the potential to enhance the cultural capital of men and women looking for secure employment. As in earlier decades, different models of femininity persisted: nurses were still influenced by the model of a dedicated, amenable gentlewoman, still the good woman, still the hand-maiden, but also the worker, the handy-woman. Nursing was, however, losing its attraction for a new middle-class educational elite, with a concomitant decline in its professional status.

Middleton (1987) and Skeggs (1997) make it clear that femininities are also differentiated in terms of sexuality. Furthermore, constructions of female sexuality are also linked to class and to discourses about the intellectual and practical. From my own experience in a single sex academic girls school during the 1960s, I am aware that nursing was not considered suitable as a career choice for girls expected to succeed in A levels. Women nurse colleagues have reinforced this view by noting how, once they had declared an intention to nurse, teachers ceased to concern themselves with their educational progression. Since nurses did not need A levels, girls with A levels should not be nurses. While academic girls cultivated an unworldly, bohemian, aesthetic and intellectual femininity to reduce male anxiety about women claiming intellectual equality, non-academic girls were free to present a more sexualised and exaggerated femininity. Middle-class girls, as the intellectual elite, distanced themselves from vulgar sexuality, thus maintaining moral superiority through sexual rather than spiritual control. Women's education was, therefore, an important part of a classificatory system between women as well as between men and women.

A romantic image of nursing can portray key components of femininity that Cixous (1980) identified as silent, static, invisible and composed. The nurse's uniform is a key feature of both the romantic and the sexualised imagery of nursing. Although the nursing uniform removes signs of the vulgar or tasteless and hence controls nurses' sexuality, the sexy nurse image is a perversion of this romantic image. Skeggs (1997) sees the ideal of femininity as a bourgeois sign and argues that 'femininity is deployed to halt losses, as a way of trying to generate some value' (p. 102). While women may construct nursing (and themselves) as essentially feminine to enhance their chances of gaining value through romance, it is male fantasies that construct nursing as sexualised, adjusting the uniform to do so.

Nurses' relationships with doctors

Although Porter (1992) has argued that, by the 1990s, gender ceased to be an important factor in relationships between doctors and nurses, Halford et al. (1997) found gender, sexuality and the politics of the body routinely affecting the relationships between nurses and doctors. In research exploring the gendering of careers and organisations in nursing, local government and banking, they found 'that the nurse–doctor relationship was routinely (hetero)sexualised and drew upon hegemonic forms of masculinity and emphasised femininity' (p. 238). The manifestations of the heterosexualised relationships ranged from friendly banter 'tinged with "Mills and Boon" type notions of romance' to senior medical staff's persistent references to nurses' bodies. One survey respondent noted,

> When doctors think they have a right to touch you, I think still that if you tend not to notice, that's good, but if you actually go into hysterics and draw attention, I think that makes you feel as bad yourself. But I don't know how many other people react to being touched, because we're all touched by doctors. But I wouldn't have said that's a big problem. It's part of everyday life, as far as I'm concerned.
>
> (pp. 239–40)

In contrast to nurse–doctor relationships, Halford et al. (1997) noted that female and male nurses used kinship discourses to help to negotiate their relationships, avoiding 'the pitfalls of heterosexualisation' (p. 237). Through familial 'subject positions' such as 'uncle', 'brother' and 'mother', male and female nurses negotiated relationships of equality and female authority, allowing men to position themselves in non-hegemonic masculine roles and women to limit the sexualisation of their femininity. Male nurses in the 1990s may thus be free to work with female nurses outside the heterosexuality project.

Men in nursing

The end of World War Two brought an influx of men into adult nursing. Some male general nurses' had worked in the forces as medical attendants (Rosen and Jones 1972) and chose to continue their work in nursing in peacetime; psychiatry, too, maintained its appeal for men after the war. Williams' (1994) small study of male voices in nursing confirmed the attraction of psychiatry. Male strength and presumed skills in control and restraint were seen as being relevant skills for the job. In addition, since large psychiatric institutions had sports facilities and football and cricket teams, an ability and interest in sport were also perceived as valuable. Williams (1994) notes that such views, coupled with the view that nursing provided a regular wage, allowed men to enter psychiatric nursing with their masculinity 'well shored up'. Nolan (1989) describes how some male psychiatric nurses with wartime experience initially found congruence between military life and nursing. Ex-soldiers found the nursing uniform, the controlling regimes and the comradeship of other ex-army nurses a supportive structure via which to readjust to civilian life (see Chapter 9).

Discriminatory practices against men in nursing were progressively removed. The 1949 Nurses Act amalgamated men onto the same register as women, the RCN accepted male members in 1960, and the Sex Discrimination Act 1975 eventually opened up midwifery and health visiting to men. Although there was an initial post-war rise in the proportion of men in nursing, however, the high percentage of 15.5 per cent in 1949 fell to 10.1 per cent in 1986, and during the 1970s and 80s the percentage remained around 10 per cent (Milligan 1993: 13).

Research into male recruitment suggests that, on average, male nurses enter nursing with lower qualifications than females as well as entering the profession later and after employment experience elsewhere. Brown and Stones (1970), in a study that involved interviewing 542 male student nurses, found that 53 per cent of student nurses and 19 per cent pupil nurses were over 21 when they started training. More recently, Marsland *et al.* (1996) analysed questionnaire responses from 936 women and 79 men qualifying as general nurses, finding that the men were slightly older than the women, were more likely to have worked in full-time employment before entering nurse education and were less likely than women to have chosen nursing as a first career option. Only 18 per cent of men said that nursing was their first choice, compared with 49 per cent of women. Although Rosen and Jones (1972) reported that men were less likely to have a grammar school education than women nurses, Marsland *et al.*

(1996) found no gender differences in educational qualification. In their study, men were more likely to say that they planned to move into education, research and management, whereas women were more likely to plan to work in the community and to aim to stay in clinical practice. Although for some men, the 'choice' of nursing may be a result of lack of academic qualifications for entry to other professions and hence influenced by their restricted career opportunities elsewhere, Ireland (1993) found that vocational and humanitarian concerns were highly significant for some men.

Men in management

Assumptions that men enter nursing for career progression developed over post-war decades during which men achieved considerable success in gaining senior positions in nurse education and management. The career progression of men in a predominantly female profession has prompted considerable comment. The Salmon Report (MoH and SHHD 1966), which recommended a managerial structure for nursing that ensured the representation of the profession at employing authority level and at all relevant levels throughout the service, was seen by some commentators as a 'male nurses' charter', containing 'uncritical approval of male values and masculine knowledge and abilities' (Austin 1977: 116). Milligan (1993), however, argues that Salmon's text is more gender neutral than such comments suggest and notes that the rise in the number of men in managerial positions considerably predated Salmon. Appendix 5 of the Salmon Report shows that, in England and Wales over the period 1960–64, 20.5 per cent of 5418 matrons/chief male nurses and deputy matrons/deputy chief males nurses were male, and of 1434 tutorial staff, 28.75 per cent were male (MoH and SHHD 1966: 134). These percentages are significant since male nurses rarely achieved senior positions prior to the 1960s, except in psychiatry. There was an overwhelming assumption that matrons would occupy the most senior nursing roles. When psychiatric hospitals were segregated by sex, the matron took precedence over the chief male nurse. It was not until sex segregation in psychiatric hospitals ended that men could compete equally with women. Lloyd correctly predicted that the broader outlook of married men, with work experience outside nursing, would be welcomed by hospital management committees, noting that such committees had begun

> to accept the idea that nursing administration is not altogether a female monopoly and that a well trained, well qualified and experienced man can bring to this field a certain stability and quality of leadership which is totally new to nursing.
>
> (Lloyd 1965: 363)

The Salmon Report pointed to the matrons' lack of managerial qualifications as a difficulty. Male managerial success increased rapidly after the implementation of the Salmon reforms. Nuttall (1983) noted that, in 1982, 43.8 per cent of all District Nursing Officer posts and 50.5 per cent of all Director of Nurse Education posts in England were held by men. Nuttall expressed concern that men at the top would continue to recruit men to the top, but also noted that the increasing number of married women in the profession meant that women nurses were adopting a very different pattern of work from that of the predominantly single female workforce of earlier decades. Hutt's (1985) study of Regional Nursing Officers and District Nursing Officers identified two distinct groups of senior nurses. The characteristics of one group were male, married with a family, relatively mobile, career minded, having worked outside the NHS and initially trained as a Registered Mental Nurse. The females in the other group were not married, mostly did not have children, had not worked outside the NHS and had initially trained as a general nurse. Neither of these two different groups were representative of the profession as a whole.

Davies and Rosser (1986) studied discrimination against women employees in the NHS. Their significant and widely quoted findings showed that whereas the average time taken for men to reach nursing officer grade from initial qualification was 8.4 years, women took, on average, 17.9 years. Women with continuous careers took 14.5 years, while women who took career breaks took 22.7 years. The difference between male and female promotion prospects was attributed to the fact that career paths within the NHS were male career paths, comprising a 'golden pathway' demanding long hours, home study, continuous service and geographical mobility. Women were disadvantaged by being unable to follow the golden pathway and were further disadvantaged by an organisational climate that was hostile to women. The skills and experience of many women in low-grade jobs were unwittingly supporting the promotion prospects of others. Davies (1995) has continued to explore the gendered nature of organisations and the invisibility of nursing's work in the context of a gendered culture that takes women's labour for granted.

Studies of men in nursing show that they and their work are visible (Evans 1997). Their visibility may make it easier to progress along the golden pathway. Ryan and Porter (1993) have suggested that, in Britain, such a pathway may include success in nurse education and nursing research. Their analysis of contributors to a UK-based international nursing journal, the *Journal of Advanced Nursing,* in the early 1990s showed that 45.1 per cent of UK-based writers were male, compared with only 5.5 per cent of North American contributors. Other British journals showed a similar overrepresentation of men among contributors.

Nurses may have difficulty disrupting the masculine influence over the knowledge project. Studies of male nurses, however, do not give clear reasons for men's success, beyond the obvious factors concerning continuous employment and more interest in promotion. Halford *et al.* (1997) found that men noted that their family responsibilities increased their career orientation, a choice rarely available to women. Male nurses report differences in their relationships with doctors, which they often perceive as easier, but reactions from patients and other nurses, as Jones found in a study exploring the social image of the male nurse, could range from 'total acceptance to total rejection' (Jones 1984: 1). Men in Halford *et al.*'s (1997) study reported that their difference led them to take considerable care in building working relationships with female colleagues and clients. Other studies have suggested that female nurses may feel that men take advantage of their novelty status or that female colleagues protect them. Ireland (1993) found that women admitted to treating male nurses as special because of their minority status.

Masculinities and nursing

Ireland's (1993) study also explores the complexity of the reasons why men enter nursing. Although the older men (aged 28–38) had worked prior to entering nurse training, not all had worked in dead end jobs from which nursing could be seen as an escape route. Several had decided to make a career change in order to find more satisfying work, showing a commitment to working with the most disadvantaged groups in learning disabilities and mental health. Young men entering nursing experienced negative reactions, including jokes about being a 'nancy boy' and being asked why they had not found something better to do. Others found that nursing was suggested to them after having failed to gain the grades necessary for another health-related profession such as physiotherapy. Dolan (1990) has suggested that men often come into nursing because it offers more emotional gain than other available work. Other studies have outlined the importance of job satisfaction and of patient contact and patient care for men in nursing (Murray and Chambers 1990, Alderton 1991). Factors that deter young boys from considering entering nursing, however, include hard work for low pay, making it difficult to support a family (Ellerby 1988, Holmes 1987). Thus, research into men's reasons for choosing to nurse suggest that the intrinsic rewards of the job are at least as important as the opportunities for promotion.

Men do, however, encounter resistance, prompted by society's gender expectations. Ireland's (1993) study compared women entering engineering with men entering nursing. She found that female engineers' identities as women were not questioned in the same way as male nurses' identities as men. Nevertheless, the fact that young men are entering nursing not just as a job, or as a job with prospects, but because of an intrinsic interest in the work and a sense of altruism, may be a significant step for both nursing and for gender relations.

If the twentieth century has been a century of change in gender relations and a century of progress for women, it is not easy to say the same for nursing. This may be because of the power of the ideological projects that are supported by particular constructions of nursing and constructions of gender. Nursing, men and women are entrapped by these projects, which are in turn embedded in daily social life. Although the public image of nursing does, as Hallam (1998) suggests, function as a discourse of femininity, the public image of nursing has often reflected a restricting construction of femininity. Hence nurse recruitment has been considerably affected, often negatively, by women's changing and widening roles. Nursing has not necessarily shown itself to be at ease with changing roles for women, or with women's diversity. For several decades from 1945, in media and recruitment literature, nurses are 'imaged as providers of support, assistance, comfort and compassion, rather than possessors of clinical expertise, knowledge skills and information' (Hallam 1998: 40). Furthermore, the romanticised and sexualised imagery of attractive young female nurses has had few contrasts 'other than the mocking image of petty authoritarianism found in some popular films' (Hallam 1998: 40).

Despite continued associations with the 'good woman' and the respectability of the morality project, nursing as a profession *used* mothers' willingness to work as a flexible, reserve labour force but did little to support mothers in the health care labour market. As a result, nursing's ability to recruit and retain intelligent and committed women fell. The need for labour to staff the NHS in support of the treatment advances made by the medical profession can be seen to have deskilled nurses, emphasising their subordinate status as women and as workers. Nevertheless, in recent decades, with increased opportunities for women being reflected in an improved educational preparation and broadening opportunities for nurses, nursing has begun to play a role in challenging gendered assumptions about knowledge. Similarly, although some men in nursing have sought management positions, others are entering the profession through concerns of responsibility and altruism – not the 'good woman' but the 'good citizen', acting in the intimate world of personal care rather than just the public world of government.

PART III

Gender, autonomy and
management

6 What do nurses do? Caring as a gendered concept

Introduction

The histories of nursing presented in Chapters 4 and 5 say little about what nurses actually did, or do. However, if the nature and intrinsic rewards of the job motivate both men and women to become and to remain nurses, but 90 per cent of nurses are female, it is obvious that the relationship between gender and the practice and rewards of nursing warrants discussion. This chapter looks at nursing as an activity and at different approaches to understanding and describing nurses' work. The relationship between nursing as women's work is explored, focusing on the importance of 'care' as a nursing activity and as an activity associated with femininity. In sociology, nursing work has been analysed as 'emotional labour' (James 1989).

Although Florence Nightingale saw cleaning and care of the physical environment as an important part of nurses' responsibilities, much of the work that nurses did in the past has now become the responsibility of domestic staff. Nurses did more than provide domestic labour, however: they provided support for medical care and they organised patients, staff and the care environment in order to ensure the smooth running of the hospital. Whereas principles of hygiene comprised an important part of nursing's knowledge in the nineteenth century, nursing curricula expanded in the twentieth century to include disease processes and principles of cure. In Britain, however, it was not until the 1970s that curricula included nurses' own analysis of the nature of nursing and nursing work. This development was heavily influenced by Henderson's (1966) analysis of the 'unique function' of the nurse. Henderson's work led to the development of nursing models and to the 'nursing process', a systematic approach to nursing care. During the 1970s, holistic models of patient care developed, portraying the nurse–patient relationship in a way that acknowledged the importance of social and psychological as well as biological influences on health and illness (Armstrong 1983, Salvage 1992). Nurses gained a new responsibility, that of understanding clients' subjective responses to their experiences. The 'New Nursing' (Salvage 1992), which comprised developments in methods of organising nursing such as primary nursing (Pearson 1988), paved the way for the increasing emphasis on equal partnerships with service users that has developed through policy initiatives since 1989 (DoH 1989a, 1989b). In addition, other writers, notably Jean Watson (1979, 1985), Patricia Benner (1984) and Benner and Wrubel (1989) sought to develop nurses' understanding of caring and argued that 'the practice of caring is central to nursing' (Watson 1979: 9).

Nursing care and the traditional image of the nurse

Watson attributed the difficulties in encouraging nurses to recognise the importance of what she called 'the science of caring in nursing' to the conflict with the traditional image of nursing. In the past, she argued, nurses as a cultural group

> were 'other directed' rather than 'inner directed'. Nursing was influenced by medical groups and the professional lives of nurses were directed by physicians. Nurses were dedicated, self-sacrificing, and deferring. They were quiet and submissive to other groups, especially to physicians. They did not question or complain; they accepted. Nurses had difficulty with authority and self-esteem... Consistent with those conditions were the philosophy and practice that the nurse learns by doing. The only way students could become nurses was to do certain jobs again and again – 'practice makes perfect'... Nurses were very much occupied with the completion of tasks, procedures, charts, physical care and management of the ward. As persons the nurses were likely to be rigid, conformist, self-controlled, self-regulated, self-composed, and highly professional – to the extent there was no expression of personal feelings and no distinction among nurses as people.
>
> (Watson 1979: 53)

Whereas Watson discusses the traditional image of the nurse in gender-neutral terms, Kuhse (1997) is clear that such an image arose through 'the cultural tradition of the nineteenth century, a tradition that gave an unequal status to women and men, and placed much emphasis on hierarchical social organisation and authoritarian lines of command' (p. 13). Although nurses' subservient role to medicine can be seen as functional, ensuring that decision making is in the hands of those with the greatest knowledge, a point argued by Newton (1981), feminist critiques suggest such subservience led to compliant, dependent nurses.

Reverby (1987a, 1987b) has argued that the conventional nineteenth century construction of women's roles and character led to women's vocation and duty to care becoming the rationale for the development of nursing as a public and professional activity. Nurses were expected to develop their skills through using and honing their natural characteristics of womanly virtue. Nursing could thus be presented as a naturally occurring activity rather than work chosen by an autonomous and self-directed agent. In order to recast our understanding of nurses' relationships with patients, nurses had to see themselves as autonomous agents, capable of acting independently in the best interests of the clients, and indeed as their advocates. It is through exploring the independent and autonomous area of nursing, as opposed to medical practice, that 'care' as opposed to 'cure' has received close attention.

Although the nursing emphasis on care has recently had a significant impact on theoretical discussions about nursing, the idea of nursing and medicine's separate spheres is not new. Nineteenth-century nurse leaders used Victorian ideas concerning the separate spheres of men and women and differences in abilities between the sexes to identify nursing's autonomous space within health care. Nineteenth century views of nursing's autonomy depended on essentialist views of the good woman. Watson (1979) has developed a taxonomy of caring, and Benner and Wrubel (1989) have explored the meaning of care through presenting detailed accounts of nursing practice. These accounts demonstrate nurses' ability to participate in the 'shared human language of emotions and lived experiences' (Bowden 1997: 108), which allow them to attune their capabilities to the client's lived experience of illness (see Chapter 10).

Care and the intrinsic rewards of nursing

It would be difficult to argue that nurses have only recently discovered 'care' and a sense of responsibility. Mackay (1989), in her substantial study, found that caring, along with commitment and character, was a taken-for-granted attribute of a 'good nurse'. The intrinsic rewards of the work were the satisfaction gained through doing 'something worthwhile'. Mackay quotes qualified and learner nurses' accounts of the satisfaction they gain from their work:

> I like looking after people. I like feeling responsibility. I like delegating work. I like the feeling when everything's gone well at the end of the shift. I suppose all that. I like the excitement when it's busy, yes. I get satisfaction out of that. (Staff Nurse)

> I like people. I like to be around people, especially people who cannot do for themselves. You know, it's just knowing you've done your good deed for the day sort of thing... I just love the old people, I think they're super. You have got so much to learn from them, no matter how 'mental' they are. (Pupil)

> (Mackay 1989: 133–4)

Enjoying 'being good', feeling responsible and feeling good about themselves was not confined to women. A charge nurse in Mackay's study commented,

> I think it's given me a feeling of self-worth... And I think I'm doing something socially useful at the end of the day.

> (p. 139)

Mackay found that a growth in confidence, self-esteem, increased tolerance and a greater awareness of others' problems were all attributes that nurses gained from their job. Many mentioned that being a nurse became an important part of their self-identity. 'It sort of gets hold of you' (enrolled nurse); 'I think you get to be addicted to it' (sister) (Mackay 1989: 135). For some, nursing is more than a job.

Developing a caring self

Whereas nursing may have gained its characteristics from nineteenth century notions of femininity, the gendered nature of caring may still mean that developing an awareness of 'a caring self' remains important as a means whereby young women develop positive self-identities. Skeggs (1997) has charted the way in which young working-class girls studying caring courses in further education came to 'recognise themselves as caring women' (p. 56). Skeggs notes that,

> For those who had already experienced the negative allocative function of the education system by the age of 16, whose employment prospects are bleak and cultural capital limited, caring (whether paid or unpaid) offers the means to value, trade and invest in themselves, an opportunity to 'make something of themselves'. It enables them to be recognised as respectable, responsible and mature...
>
> To be a caring person involves having to display responsibility by taking on personality traits such as unselfishness. Responsibility as one of the key signifiers of respectability is demonstrated through self-performances, such as conduct and manners, or through the care and obligations to others (for example familial, voluntary and occupational caring). The caring self is a dialogic production: a caring self cannot be produced without caring for others.
>
> (1997: 56)

However, for many young women, the decision to take a caring course may be not so much a positive decision as an attempt to gain a cultural resource through 'something at which they are unlikely to fail' (Skeggs 1997: 58) and within a restricted range of choices. Skeggs notes the relevance of the views expressed by Connell *et al.* (1982), which suggest that caring qualifications may be a form of cultural capital that prevents individuals from further cultural and economic slippage. Caring courses already have the lowest status in the college hierarchy, a hierarchy that is 'premised on the sexual division of labour which divides students on the basis of their previous gendered and classed educational capital'. Thus, for the young women,

> Not only are the courses entered by default, they are entered with a clear awareness of distinctions. Eventually the women come to invert their differences by stressing the practical side of their courses over the uselessness of academic qualifications. This can be seen as the beginning of a process lived throughout their lives in which they attempt to gain some status and value for themselves through their cultural capital in the face of negation.
>
> (Skeggs 1997: 59)

Unsurprisingly, therefore, a stage in the young women's nego-tiation of the caring course is what Skeggs terms 'celebrating the practical', particularly the occupationally related practical work, at the expense of the academic side of the curriculum: 'A caring self is a practical, not academic self' (p. 59). Skeggs makes use of Donald's (1985) argument that the curriculum establishes hierar-chical relationships between different forms of knowledge that generate subject positions in relation to the hierarchies; 'for example, it defines what it is to be cultivated and clever against what it is to be practical, useful and responsible. These subject positions provide character definitions' (p. 60). Through their experiences in the practical side of the caring course, the young women came to see themselves as caring individuals. A key element in this process was the responsibility that they were sometimes forced to demonstrate in their placements:

> There I was left on my own in this hospital ward, just me, everyone else had gone, for tea or something, and there were all the medicines to be given. They'd told me to give them out, by myself, measuring milligrams. I was ever so careful and I did it.
>
> (Theresa, quoted in Skeggs 1997: 60)

Through placements, students perceived themselves as having a caring personality and caring characteristics; they were often encouraged to see themselves as 'made for the job', their caring characteristics being described as 'natural'. Through the course, their caring capabilities are open to scrutiny and their varied place-ments could throw doubt on previous caring experiences. 'The women are encouraged to develop and monitor responsibilities through their own assessment of good and bad caring practice' (Skeggs 1997: 65). Skeggs found that, in Florence Nightingale tradition, 'hygiene is a strong signifier of respectability *and* of good caring practice' (p. 65) – but so is selflessness, and the necessity continually to prove themselves through the course assessments and through their caring performances for others threatens their positive self-evaluation. Their achievement of respectability and responsibility is at potentially great cost to themselves, the cost of a continuous self-monitoring.

The significance of Skeggs' work for nursing is clear. Her analysis of learning to care suggests that it is not so much that 'good women' are selected for their caring qualities, but that the practice experience of caring allows women to recognise their caring attributes and thereby create a self-identity that claims caring as an unlearned characteristic. Skeggs' work suggests that although the theoretical content of the caring courses also provides knowledge that fosters a more critical awareness of caring practices, it is the responsibility of caring for others that constructs the respectability of the good woman as much as the recruitment of good women that constructs the respectability of caring work. Whereas nursing brought young *middle-class* nineteenth-century women an opportunity to gain experience beyond their domestic world, in the late twentieth century, caring courses in further education bring a similar opportunity to young *working-class* girls.

There is no reason to assume that men cannot find equal satisfaction in the development and recognition of caring responsibility as a personal attribute: male nurses provide evidence that they do. Excluding men from caring responsibility, however, serves to reinforce a range of masculinities that support a variety of ideological projects – the heterosexual project, the knowledge project, the capitalism project. If men are heterosexual predators, active decision makers, abstract thinkers, their concern must be the bourgeois individualistic concern for care of the self rather than care for others. Freedom lies in the autonomous self. As Skeggs notes, in bourgeois individualist practice, 'it is the prerogative of someone who does not have to care for others to be seen as worthy of respect' (1997: 64). Women rarely have this prerogative and thus earn their respectability through their care for others, but it is a respectability, judged through a standard of individual autonomy and decision making, that is devalued in a culture stratified by class and gender as well as along other dimensions.

Gaining knowledge about care

Unsurprisingly, explorations of care and of processes of learning to care are forced to deal with epistemological questions. Skeggs found that when the women in her study were asked to describe what caring involved, they answered in terms of the personality dispositions they saw as essential to caring – kind and loving, considerate about others, understanding. The descriptions were,

Skeggs argues, enunciated in terms of 'wider discourses of how women should be'. Intuition, defined as both instinctive and a product of experience, was seen as 'the ultimate caring disposition' and as a feminine mental aptitude (Skeggs 1997: 69). Benner (1984) has described intuition as a mode of cognition that characterises expert nursing practice.

Watson (1979) attempted to identify a scientific knowledge base for nursing's humanistic value system, arguing that an integration of knowledge from the biophysical and behavioural sciences with the humanities would provide a basis for the development of carative factors. As such, she could be seen as attempting to include knowledge about care in a masculinist knowledge project. Benner and Wrubel (1989), however, have concentrated specifically on the phenomenological exploration of subjective experiential feelings and the ways in which nurses make use of their own experiential knowledge to make connections with the cared-for's lived experience of illness. They argue that a committed, involved stance allows carer and cared-for to share emotions arising from the existential dilemmas of health and illness. For Benner and Wrubel, 'caring is always specific and relational', and therefore no 'context-free' prescriptions can guide all caring practices (1989: 3). In sociology, Fox (1993) has drawn on postmodernism in formulating his analysis of care. From this standpoint, knowledge is constructed through discourse, and discourses construct subjectivities. Power is linked to knowledge (Foucault 1980), and care practices founded on knowledge deriving from generalised theories of care can lead to, in Fox's terms, 'care-as-discipline', a possessive and controlling 'vigil of care' (Fox 1993, 1995). It is the care professions that create controlling discourses of care. The vigil is about power. Following Foucault's analysis, however, Fox argues that resistance to the disciplinary nature of care is possible. Through the everyday, individual practices of care between carer and cared-for, 'it is possible to resist the vigil of care' and to enact, in continued opposition to care-as-discipline, 'a different kind of "care" which celebrates difference and is mediated by love, generosity, trust and delight – *a gift of care*' (1995: 108).

Bowden (1997), writing from a philosophical tradition, uses Wittgenstein's approach to conceptual clarification to explore the nature of caring. She emphasises the value of 'perspicuity' (Wittgenstein 1958: 122) formed through 'a discerning juxtaposition of different "objects of comparison" that enables appropriate connections to be made among them' (Bowden 1997: 13). Bowden juxtaposes accounts of mothering, friendship, nursing and citizenship as ethical practices in order to consider the ethical nature of caring.

Despite differences in methods, most writers adopt qualitative approaches to the study of care, emphasising the perspectival, context-dependent character of both their theories and descriptions of care. They identify care in the detail of attentiveness and response that is context specific, related to particular individuals, integrating bodily activities, emotion and, in Benner's (1984) term, 'discretionary judgement'. Knowledge for care, therefore, is context specific and hence difficult to incorporate into a 'masculine' (or modernist) project seeking universal knowledge.

Gender, care and ethics

The view that there is a moral dimension to care is familiar to nursing's history and to current debates concerning care. The ethical aspects of care have been extensively discussed since Carol Gilligan's (1982) significant work addressing the possibility of a 'different voice' from the 'masculine voice' of universalist values that dominated philosophical analysis. Gilligan's ideas developed through years of research listening to children talk about moral issues. She postulated that there were two different ethical approaches at work, one based on justice, the other on the logic of care. Davies links the two ethics to cultural codes of gender:

> On the one hand there is an 'ethics of justice'; this involves a clear sense that a person is autonomous, has rights and must act responsibly, that is by following a set of formal rules of behaviour, but in essence pursues self-development. On the other hand, there is an 'ethics of care', where concern for others overrides personal autonomy, responsibilities are more important than rights and altruism and self-sacrifice are important. The first can appear from the vantage point of the second as pure selfishness; the second can appear from the vantage point of the first as dependency and indecisiveness.
>
> (1995: 27)

Gilligan's work has promoted considerable debate, particularly concerning the extent to which different modes of reasoning are associated with different genders. As Kuhse (1997) notes, this idea is not new. Rousseau (1966) distinguished between male and female virtues, arguing that female virtues flourish in the privacy of the home. Rousseau saw women's reasoning as being different, requiring systematising by men:

> The search for abstract and speculative truth, for principles and axioms of science, for all that tends to wide generalisation, is beyond a woman's grasp; their studies should be thoroughly practical. It is their business to apply the principles discovered by men.
>
> (1966: 340)

Although Gilligan characterised the different voice by theme rather than by gender, her work can be seen as giving greater emphasis to the importance of the practical, relational and partial nature of caregiving. Empirical links between women and the voice of care are generally explained through the link between the work women do and the moral concerns they raise. The danger of biological essentialist interpretations have been noted and essentialist arguments have been rejected, but the debate has stimulated attempts to explore the ethical possibilities and limitations of caring practices. Bowden's exploration draws on Benner's (1984) work that identifies excellence in nursing practice. Bowden suggests that there are ethical possibilities in quality in caregiving (Bowden 1997: 105). Fox has acknowledged that the creative and altruistic potential of 'care-as-gift' is similar to the Christian view of love (Fox 1995).

Despite exploring the excellence and potential of care, both Fox and Bowden place their reviews in the context of negative perceptions of care and the controlling and inhibiting settings in which care takes place. Fox draws on the work of the feminist post-structuralist Cixous (1986), who writes about two realms: the 'Gift' and the 'Proper'. She 'opposes *Gift* relationships (which she sees as feminine) with the masculine realm of the *Proper*: of property, propriety, possession, identity and dominance' (Fox 1995: 116). Fox describes care-as-discipline as grounded in the Proper, characterised by control, surveillance and the fabrication of, rather than the response to, individual identities. Institutionalised health and social care (care-as-discipline) has often been perceived as disabling and disempowering by its recipients.

Bowden adopts a 'gender-sensitive' approach to her exploration of care, wishing to identify and acknowledge the effects of women's subordinate status on the values placed on caring practices and the consequences for carer and cared for. Noting key themes in the historical development of nursing – the sexual division of labour, the hierarchical organisation of labour and training, the emphasis on duty and obedience, the need for cheap and willing workers, and the submission of female autonomy to male medical and managerial authority – she suggests that

> the historical consolidation of nurses' obedience to authoritarian demands, has largely thwarted their claims and capacities to define their own practice. The nexus of formal knowledge, authority and institutional control has characteristically overwhelmed the claims of personal, experiential and responsive caring that are so central to ethical excellence in nursing.
>
> (Bowden 1997: 139–40)

A gender-sensitive approach to ethics involves an awareness of the sociopolitical context in which definitions of skill and of ethical practices take place. It is such an approach that has fuelled the criticisms of the ethics of justice approach, which seeks to resolve dilemmas in terms of universal principles concerning rights, duties and autonomy. 'Justice' approaches emphasise the necessity of impartiality in decision making. Relationships become impersonal and interchangeable, in contrast to the responsive and attentive flexibility necessary for care (care-as-gift). The relationship characteristic of a justice approach is that of the citizen's relationship to the state. A gender-sensitive approach, however, would acknowledge that women have been denied full citizenship rights in many societies and many epochs. It is thus male reasoning that emphasises ethical approaches based on universalist principles. The importance of these principles is sustained through political and philosophical education in an educational system (the Academy) that itself emphasises the value of abstract analysis over and above knowledge grounded in experience and practice.

Feminist critiques of the political construction of citizenship recognise the importance of reconstructing citizenship to take account of men's and women's diversity and difference. Lister (1997) seeks to refashion the yardstick of universalism

> so that the universal and the particular are combined in an unbiased way: a differentiated instead of a false universalism.

A key issue in the refashioning of the yardstick is the value to be placed upon care for citizenship and the recognition of care as a political ideal and practice that transcends the public–private divide.

(p. 200)

Lister identifies the necessity to formulate policies that take account of *all* citizens as citizen the earner/carer: to distinguish between citizen as earner and citizen as carer would disadvantage women by further confining them to caring roles. Bowden (1997), writing from a different starting point (philosophy rather than social policy), has suggested that community care policies are the means by which caring practices can become part of the responsibilities of citizens. As she notes, however, 'the use of the language of care in discussions of the values of citizenship is frequently dismissed as reactionary – as damaging to the cause of women's equality, drawing on inappropriate relational models and appealing to the whims of particularised compassion' (Bowden 1997: 160).

Social science analyses of care

In Britain, social scientists have been quick to note the possible damage to the cause of women's equality that may result from community care policies (DoH 1989a). Finch and Groves (1983) argued that community care policies were incompatible with equal opportunities for women since assumptions concerning women's care for older and disabled people would limit women's opportunities to participate in the labour market. Studies exploring women's role in informal care (Ungerson 1987, Lewis and Meredith 1988) played a valuable part in highlighting the gendered nature of care and served as a critique of policy. However, the emphasis on women's role in the labour market also served to narrow the focus of social science study concerning care, to the extent that women's role in childcare and women's role as paid carers became excluded from the debate. Furthermore, disabled women identified that academic feminists had ignored the interests of women in receipt of care (Morris 1993). In seeking to ensure that the rights of able-bodied, employable women were not curtailed, 'the feminist caring literature had treated disabled people as themselves invisible, passive, homogeneous and dependent'

(Ungerson 1997: 345). Dalley (1988) and Finch (1990) both went as far as to espouse residential care for the older and disabled people in need of care. Morris (1993) made the point that

> Undoubtedly, the generally prejudicial attitudes towards older and disabled people – which undermine their human and civil rights – had an important influence on the ability of feminists such as Finch and Dalley to feel that a denial of a home and family life were appropriate social reactions to growing older or experiencing physical, sensory or intellectual impairment.
>
> (p. 47)

Morris makes it clear that the emphasis on the economic interests of non-disabled women acted as a limitation on feminists' ability to recognise the interests of older and disabled people. Feminist literature, however, has placed such neglect of the diversity of women's needs and interests in the context of a more widespread failure of 1970s feminism to identify difference. Care research had also ignored the effect of class and race on diversity of caregiving practices and had underestimated the extent to which men were involved in care. The 1985 General Household Survey asked questions designed to identify carers, the results of this survey indicating that 11 per cent of men reported caring obligations, compared with 15 per cent women. The extent of male involvement in care had been unexpected. Furthermore, the extent to which spouses undertook caring responsibilities had been underestimated, many of the older generation preferring to support each other and hence remain independent of their children (Arber and Gilbert 1989, Parker 1990).

The emphasis on informal carers also ignored paid carers, particularly nurses. The analysis of care focused largely on who provided what type of informal care and for whom. The nature of care has been analysed in terms of activity state (work, tasks, labour) and feeling state (emotion, affection, love). The difference between the activity state 'caring for' and the feeling state 'caring about' has been conceptualised as the difference between 'labour' and 'love'. Graham (1983) criticised social policy literature for ignoring the dual nature of care and concentrating on the analysis of care as labour, but her own analyses of labour and love concentrated on the private domestic setting, ignoring the public domain.

Emotional labour, emotion work and feeling rules

In sociological literature, the labour and feeling involved in nursing care has been analysed as emotional labour (James 1989), often drawing on Hochschild's (1983) work. Hochschild uses the term 'emotional labour' to mean 'the management of feeling to create a publicly observable facial and bodily display; emotional labour is sold for a wage and therefore has *exchange value*' (p. 7). Emotional labour involves managing one's own and others' feelings. Hochschild explored the emotional labour of air hostesses and debt collectors, noting the way in which their emotional labour becomes a commodity. Hochschild also uses the terms 'emotion work' and 'emotion management' to refer to the same acts of feeling management in the private setting, a setting in which they have use value rather than exchange value in an economic sense. Emotion work, however, clearly has exchange value in an interpersonal context and in interpersonal exchange. Hochschild's distinctions have been used inconsistently in the sociological literature. James, for example, has used emotional labour as a term for both domestic and public domains, seeing the setting as affecting the form of emotional labour:

> Emotional labour is organised and managed both in the private domain of home and the public domain of the workplace. The forms it takes are affected by the dominant organisation so that the form of emotional labour within the relatively pliable routines in the home differs from that which is possible within the rigidity of workplace organisation.
>
> (1989: 29)

James identifies emotional labour in both private and public settings as women's work, noting that the devaluing of the work involved in emotion management stems from the way in which 'emotion is held to contrast with rational' (p. 37), and the exclusion of emotion from the workplace. The denial of skill involved in emotional labour derives from the view that

> because emotions belong at home, they are women's work and unskilled. The contradictions mean that although women may be employed on the basis of their skills in dealing with other people's feelings, they are given no credit for those skills.
>
> (James 1989: 37)

James, a nurse and sociologist, has used the concept of emotional labour to explore the management of feelings involved in nurses' work in a hospice setting. Smith (1992) has also used the term to explore nurses' work. In addition, James (1992a, 1992b) explores the fusion of activity, feeling and organisation in the practice of care. She has noted that nurses themselves talk about 'work' as 'physical activity, doing things' (1992a: 107) as distinct from 'care', and has suggested the use of the term 'carework' as a means of helping us to understand the 'demands of emotional labour relative to physical labour', while keeping care and work as 'antagonistically separate – as thesis and antithesis' (p. 111). A further exploration of the organisational constraints has led to James' analysis of care as comprising organisation + physical labour + emotional labour, thus clarifying the importance of both the organisational context of nursing care and the importance of nurses' organisation of their own physical work in facilitating effective care (1992b). As yet, however, it is nursing literature rather than sociology that has explored the importance of what Benner and Wrubel term 'the skilled habitual body' in care (1989: 394). The neglect of practical activity and caring in academic analysis should, however, not be seen as surprising. A lack of interest in practical work has been an important part of the socialisation of academic women. Caring has been at the bottom of the educational hierarchy.

Nevertheless, in sociology, the growth in the study of emotion is fostering a literature that provides ways of thinking about health and social care. Lee Treweek (1996), for example, has explored the way in which care assistants in a residential home used emotion work to help to maintain order within the home. She uses Hochschild's term 'emotion work' rather than 'emotional labour' in order to avoid the connotations of enforced emotional behaviour' (p. 116). Much of the care assistants' emotion work was self-generated, thus bringing the care assistants an autonomous sphere of activity. Emotion work involved both nurture and control:

> The use of emotion work had a pattern or set of patterns and these were used by the assistants to define, organise and react to resident behaviour. Residents who breached the emotional order were negatively typified by both staff and other residents as a matter of course. Second,

emotion work appeared to be a strategy which empowered the women
workers as it provided an effective means of ordering the residents.

(Lee Treweek 1996: 130)

Such control of the emotional order was probably a familiar
strategy adopted by the nineteenth century good woman as good
nurse. The importance of emotion work is now being recognised in
many organisational settings. Goleman (1998), for example, has
identified the importance of emotional intelligence in management,
making reference to Hochschild's work. He suggests, however, that
a nurses' emotional labour is not perceived as onerous but as 'what
makes her job more meaningful' (Goleman 1998: 81).

Sociological research into health, illness and health care now
demonstrates a growing awareness of the importance of emotion
as experienced by both the fieldworker and the research participants. Young and Lee (1996) review a fieldworker's emotional
responses to interviews with respondents with a terminal illness in
terms of another of Hochschild's concepts, that of 'feeling rules' –
social guidelines that influence how we feel. Young and Lee
observe that the fieldworker, and nurses who facilitated the
research, responded differently to the situations encountered.
Unlike the fieldworker, the nurses 'had a response to this situation
based on their own profession's feeling rules and could do the
emotion work required' (p. 110). Young is not the only fieldworker to find that it is the emotions associated with fieldwork
that prompt an analysis of emotion work. Webb (1998), for
example, acknowledges that his own feeling of 'there but for the
grace of God' led to his analysis of the psychodynamics of care
between traumatic brain injured people and their carers. Carers,
however, do the emotion work required.

Summary

Throughout this chapter, varied views of care have been identified.
The duty to care has been seen as a woman's natural vocation;
caring has been seen as a taken-for-granted attribute of a good
nurse, and a caring self as a source of self-esteem for both nurses
and other young women on caring courses. Care is seen as a
possible gift, as a virtue, but also as a means of control. Care

represents 'a different voice' upholding feminine cultural codes with an emphasis on responsibility to others. Women's responsibilities for care have been seen as constraining and controlling women by denying them equal opportunities in the labour market. In the workplace, caring activities, defined as emotional labour and emotion work, are unrecognised and unrewarded because they are seen as women's natural skills, emanating from the domestic sphere. The skill and complexity of caregiving, involving organisation, physical activity and the management of emotion, is, however, beginning to be explored, perhaps as a necessary precursor to being valued.

There is broad agreement that care is a gendered concept in that it is associated with women and with women's work. Functionalists see it as supportive of and developed through women's role in the family, wherein it is constructed as natural, unlearned and without skill. As such, emotional labour, like domestic labour, is unpaid but nevertheless contributes to the capitalist system by maintaining the health and welfare of the workforce. In addition, emotional labour becomes a commodity to be sold within service industries. A patriarchal control of both women and the economy can be facilitated through the commercialisation and commodification of women's bodies and women's caring smiles. For some women, however, their 'caring self' is both a source of self-worth and a means of cultural capital that maintains a position, albeit lowly, in the status hierarchy. Skilled emotion work, however, can, through managing the emotional order and developing the feeling rules, be a means of control.

Care is, however, not just an attribute of the carer, but also the substance of a relationship. Care is enabling or controlling only in a relational, dialogic sense. Whereas within a patriarchal system, the view that care is gendered and the gender is feminine allows care to be denigrated and ignored, and carers blamed or taken for granted, as gender inequalities lessen, both carer and cared-for are likely to pay more attention to care.

The involvement of both men and women in professional care relationships that take the user's experience and perspective seriously could accelerate change in gendered cultural constructions.

7 Dependence, autonomy and professional roles

Introduction

Chapter 6 has already indicated the variety of processes through which caring, as an other-directed activity, acquires low status within contemporary society. This chapter links gender, emotional labour and social status to analyses of professional relationships between doctors and nurses, and to discourses about individual autonomy and identity. First, however, it looks at gender and caring relationships through accounts of the development of gendered personalities.

Gender and the development of individual identity

As Busfield (1996) makes clear, feminist theorising about gender and psychology has been significantly influenced by Freud's analysis of the power of unconscious desires, the importance of early childhood experiences and the origin of conflicts and tensions within the individual. Although Freud (1973) has been strongly criticised, notably by Millett (1972) for suggesting a relationship between female personality and the lack of a penis, followers of Freud, such as Melanie Klein (1946), have made significant contributions to interpretations of gendered development.

Klein's work contributed to the development of object relations theory in psychoanalysis. In this theory, children's perceptions of the external world and of external objects are shaped by their internal 'objects' and internal 'object-relations', which are fantasies of external reality. The external world and the inner world of object relations continually interact. Children begin life experiencing a unity with parental caregivers but progressively develop an internal world of object relations in which they make sense of themselves as individuals separate from others in the external world. The sense of self develops through relations with the external caregiver. As language and motor skills develop, a phase of separation/individuation occurs, and the child develops ways of coping with the anxiety of variations in the caregiver's response to the child's needs. Children may cope with perceived inadequacies in a carer's response by creating idealised fantasy object relations in which the carer can do no wrong. An alternative to idealisation may be rejection, based on the child's fantasy of independence. Self-blame and guilt may be another response to the need to explain any perceived neglect on the part of the caregiver. A toddler begins to recognise him or her self as a boy or a girl while recognising him or her self as a separate individual with boundaries and agency. Since a child's mother is usually the most important external object in a child's life, object relations differ for boys and girls. Within the mother–daughter relationship, the daughter must be able both to identify with her mother and also to perceive herself and her mother as separate subjectivities. Chodorow (1978) argues that because mothers experience boys as 'a male opposite' who will have social roles different from their own 'female' roles, boys more readily develop a separate, autonomous, agentic self.

Susie Orbach (1998 [1978]) has drawn on ideas concerning gender development and object relations to explore the relationship between body size and the social construction of gender through role expectations. In *Fat is a Feminist Issue*, she argues thus:

> For a mother, a crucial part of the maternal role is to help her daughter, as her mother did before her, to make a smooth transition into the female social role...

> But the world the mother must present to her daughter is one of unequal relationships, between parent and child, authority and powerlessness, man and woman. The child is exposed to the world of power relationships by a unit that itself produces and reproduces perhaps the most fundamental of these inequalities. Within the family, an inferior sense of self is instilled into little girls. While it is obvious that the growing-up process for girls and boys is vastly different, what may be less apparent is that to prepare her daughter for a life of inequality, the mother tries to hold back her child's desires to be a powerful, autonomous self-directed, energetic and productive human being. From an early age, the young girl is encouraged to accept this rupture in her development and is guided to cope with this loss by putting her energy into care of others. Her own needs for emotional support and growth will be satisfied if she can convert them into giving to others.

> (Orbach 1998 [1978]: 28–9)

This analysis of the effect of a mother's caring role on her daughter's identity has been criticised both for its dependence on roles as an explanation for gender differentiation and for the implicit generalisations that deny the diversity of women's lives. Davies (1995), however, argues that feminine cultural codes link selfless-ness and responsibility to others with connected and relational self-development. This form of self-development may stand in opposition to a masculine separation and boundedness. From this standpoint, caring, as an other-directed activity, therefore, operates according to a feminine cultural code and may inhibit the agentic autonomy of both carer and cared-for (see also Chapter 10). Although mothers and daughters may be the main example of such a process, male carers and carers in public as well as private arenas may face similar issues. As will be seen later, Davies argues for a new professionalism to enable nurses, as carers, to develop relationships in health care that are neither autonomous nor dependent but inter-dependent, and neither self-orientated nor self-effacing but 'accepting of an embodied use of self as part of a therapeutic encounter' (Davies 1995: 149–50). Similarly, it is the physical care by an autonomous parent that brings the safe environment in which an experiencing, agentic and non-dependent self develops.

It is important to note, however, that the theorists mentioned are all analysing the development of self and gendered cultural codes from a twentieth century Western standpoint. Anthropolo-gists have identified very different conceptions of self in different cultures. Geertz (1993) noted that in Java, a perception of the 'self' as having independent inner and outer realms shaped individuals' lives. Kondo (1990), a Japanese-American anthropologist who studied kinship, economics and family businesses in Tokyo, found that her research strongly challenged her Western assumptions about the boundedness of identity. Japanese women would have considerable difficulty in distinguishing between identity and context, and would perceive their personal development and maturity as inextricable from their accommodation to the duties of their status and to the needs of others. Billington *et al.* (1998), in commenting on research into different cultural conceptions of self-hood note that 'what is normal healthy and mature in one culture may be abnormal sick or immature in another' (p. 49). In Japan, a dutiful self would be a mature self. In Western culture, maturity is more closely linked with self-development than other-orientation.

Gender and emotional labour

Hochschild (1983) sees the association between women and emotional labour as deriving from the importance of women's functional roles in childcare and from their economic position, rather than from girls' identity development. Hochschild explores the status and class-based nature of emotional management. It is middle-class jobs that involve work with people. Middle-class parents engaged in emotional labour in management, service and professional jobs prepare their children in similar skills. However, since it is women more than men who work with people in their jobs, the value of emotion work is lowered through women's subordinate status. In comparison to men, Hochschild saw women as a subordinate social stratum because they have 'far less independent access to money, power, authority or status in society' (1983: 163). Hochschild identified four consequences of such social subordination:

1. 'Lacking other resources, women make a resource out of feeling and offer it to men as a gift in return for the more material resources they lack' (p. 163). Thus, relational work and emotional labour are an important resource for women, which may help to explain women's own readiness to claim caring as a (female) gendered attribute.

2. The specialisation of emotional labour according to gender rests on stereotypical assumptions about childhood socialisation in which passivity is encouraged in girls while aggression is tolerated in boys. Hence, at work, 'women are more likely to be presented with the task of mastering anger and aggression in the service of "being nice". To men, the socially assigned task of aggressing against those that break the rules of various sorts creates the private task of mastering fear and vulnerability' (Hochschild 1983: 163). Male nurses would, perhaps, concur that their behaviour is affected by gendered expectations to appear in control and indeed to exert control in situations that might threaten the health and life of themselves and others.

3. 'The general subordination of women leaves every individual woman with a weaker "status shield" against the displaced feelings of others' (Hochschild 1983: 163). In Hochschild's

study of flight attendants, it was the females who were more frequently verbally abused by passengers; male colleagues were called upon 'to handle unwarranted aggression'.

4. Gendered expectations mean that 'for each gender a different portion of the managed heart is enlisted for commercial use' (p. 164). Women feel estranged from the 'feminine' attributes that are exploited for commercial gain, that is, from their sexual beauty, charm and relational skills. Men feel estranged from the 'masculine' capacity for dominance – 'the capacity to wield anger and make threats' – that is part of their expected emotion work.

Both men and women in caring roles are, therefore, using as cultural capital, their masculinity and femininity. At the same time, however, when their gendered attributes are used as emotional labour, they can experience a sense of alienation from their commodified body. They can experience gender estrangement.

Hochschild's analysis confirms the mechanisms whereby emotional labour, despite constituting a resource for women, confirms and compounds women's subordinate status. She claims that the emotional and social work that women do is that of 'affirming, enhancing, and celebrating the wellbeing and status of others... the adaptive, co-operative women is actively working at showing deference' (Hochschild 1983: 165).

Health care professions demand considerable willingness to enhance the wellbeing of others. The skills which Hochschild suggested that women cultivated through emotion work, such as 'sensitivity to non-verbal communication and to the micropolitical significance of feeling' (p. 167), resulting in a skilled capacity to get things done, seemingly effortlessly, are intrinsic to health care. Unseen, the emotional labour, like housework, is unrecognised and unrewarded. Used in the promotion of others' worth, it is seen as deference and dismissed as an attribute of the subordinate:

> Women accommodate, then, but not passively. They adapt feeling to a need or a purpose at hand, and they do it so that it seems to express a passive state of agreement, a chance occurrence of coinciding needs. Being becomes a way of doing. Acting is the needed art, and emotion work is the tool.
>
> (Hochschild 1983: 167)

Emotional labour, perhaps, is the work that makes a good woman a good nurse (or the gentleman a good citizen). Yet, despite emphasising the relationship between women and emotional labour, Hochschild is clear that the increasing use of emotional labour in commercial and service settings is a phenomenon of American culture that affects men and women. An emphasis on the social uses of feeling in any system of mass production leaves those performing emotional labour at risk of seeing 'a smile, a mood, a feeling, or a relationship as belonging more to the organisation and less to the self' (Hochschild 1983: 198).

Caring, subservience and autonomy

Several questions emerge from the above analyses of, first, the potential of the mother–daughter relationship to create dependency in adult female personalities, and second, the importance of emotion work among subordinate social strata, particularly women. Do other-directed caring relationships necessarily reduce autonomous agency of the individual carer – male or female – and confine caring professions to a subordinate status? Do women carers find it more difficult than male carers to avoid exploitation, subservience and acquiescence in caring roles? If so, are there significant consequences for those they care for? Is cultural change, including changing gender roles, facilitating changing conceptions of care and increasing the recognition of the importance of emotional labour? If the last question can be answered in the affirmative, nurses have opportunities to participate in and promote significant social change.

Emotional labour and the doctor–nurse relationship

Stein's (1967) seminal analysis of the doctor–nurse relationship as the doctor–nurse game demonstrates nurses' use of emotional labour to influence health care decisions. Stein described the object of the game, which he presented as common in the 1960s, as:

the nurse is to be bold, have initiative, and be responsible for making significant recommendations, while at the same time she must appear passive. This must be done in such a manner so as to make her recommendations appear to be initiated by the physician.

(1967: 699)

The rules of the game are that disagreement must be avoided at all cost. The nurse communicates the recommendation without appearing to; the doctor asks for a recommendation without appearing to. The context of the game was the nature of medical training through which fear of making a mistake, coupled with the need to be seen to exercise authority and to make decisions, led to unwarranted certainty and feelings of omnipotence, making it impossible to ask for advice. The strict discipline of nurse training, on the other hand, led to respect for doctors, fear of independent action and fear of making a mistake. A learned sense of responsibility for the patient, however, led to the development of the game. Through such a game, which is largely dependent on nurses' emotional labour involved in deference work, both sides can win. Through the alliances and teamwork generated, each gains respect for the other profession.

Further studies observing doctor–nurse interactions have suggested that although the doctor–nurse game is still enacted, nurses are now more assertive in making suggestions to, or in challenging, medical colleagues. Hughes (1988) found that nurses were prepared to be openly assertive in an accident and emergency department. Porter (1992) recorded successful assertive challenges to doctors' requests in an intensive care unit. Mackay (1993), however, reporting on a study of relationships between nurses and doctors, carried out in five locations in England and Scotland from 1989 to 1990, found variations in relationships. Factors that influenced the doctor–nurse relationship included the grades of the participants, the length of time over which the relationship had developed and the experience of the nurse. Mackay notes that

whether nurses are new to their post, whether their opinion or views are to be trusted, whether they offer the information in the 'right way', whether they are forceful in offering their opinions are some of the variables affecting the extent to which nurses are listened to.

(1993: 174)

Some nurses demonstrated an awareness of the importance of finding the 'right way':

> The nurses feel they have to phrase it in a certain way instead of just saying 'why don't you use A', they'll say 'the last time this patient was in they used drug A and they found the patient much better on that and I was wondering if possibly...' and they go through this whole rigmarole of taking three times as long to get to the same point because you know that if you suggest it....

> (Sister, quoted in Mackay 1993: 173)

Mackay's report suggests that it is senior doctors who benefit overall from the emotion work and game playing of their subordinates. Some consultants see themselves as relatively free from the constraints of emotional control, seeing themselves as a 'senior person enjoying the privilege of being able to be ill tempered at times when other people are bound to suppress it...' (consultant, quoted in Mackay 1993: 177). Hence freedom from, or expectations in, emotion work have been related to hierarchical status. Mackay is critical of nurses for their silence and their acquiescence, noting that nurses viewed the medical profession with awe or subservience and doctors shared a view of nurses' subordinate status. A lack of understanding of each other's roles and workload contributed to some negative assumptions about the two professions. Mackay (1995), in a further commentary on the research findings, suggests that the doctor–nurse game may only be enacted during junior house officers' first weeks on medical and surgical wards. Despite acknowledging that some nurses do seek to challenge medical dominance, Mackay argues most are silent, engaging in performances that 'reduce the confidence of nurses in their own independent action' and as such are active in maintaining medical power and nurses' subordination (Mackay 1995: 358).

Mackay (1993) suggests that the gendered nature of nursing and medicine as occupations limits the significance of male nurses and female doctors as change agents. Women doctors adopt a scientific and rational view of medicine, and male nurses, although often mistaken for doctors, find their status affected by stereotypical views of the male nurse as gay or effeminate. Porter, however, argued that the refusal of many nurses to acquiesce without objection to the subordinate position that some doctors expected them to take... were predicated upon an increasingly positive self-evaluation of nurses about their role as female workers... In addition, the increasing proportion of female doctors seems to be leading to an attenuation of gender as a factor in nurse–doctor power relations.

(1992: 524)

Stein, in revisiting the doctor–nurse game, also found that 'one of the players (the nurse) has unilaterally decided to stop playing the game and instead is consciously and actively attempting to change' (Stein *et al.* 1990: 547).

Autonomy and professional projects

Walby *et al.* (1994) have argued that the difference between doctors' and nurses' success, or lack of it, in gaining managerial roles in health care Trusts related to differences in doctors' and nurses' emphasis on individual autonomy. Medicine had developed as a profession emphasising the importance of abstract knowledge and individual autonomy and expertise. Nursing, on the other hand, had developed as a hierarchically organised, rule-bound occupation, playing a supportive and subordinate role to medicine (Porter 1999). Davies (1995) argues that medicine's professionalism, indeed the very concept of a profession, is gendered, shaped through a culture dominated by masculine cultural codes, which can be seen as supporting the masculine 'knowledge project'. Professions sustain a 'masculine vision' through the processes that develop expertise. Professional expertise is based on a 'formalised training based on science', acquired

by dint of a lengthy and heroic effort. This effort is a project involving mastery, resulting in knowledge as a 'possession' of the autonomous individual. Knowledge and associated skills and techniques are exercised in a visible, tangible and agentic way to 'make a difference in the world'.

(Davies 1995: 59)

The autonomous professional acts according to universal values, employing skills impartially and therefore without emotion. Davies (1995) notes that 'autonomy stands at the very heart of both cultural concepts of masculinity and professions' (p. 60). We could also add that autonomy stands at the heart of Western cultural concepts of identity. The portrayal of professional autonomy, however, is only possible through misrepresenting or ignoring the work of others, as, indeed, in the doctor–nurse game, in which nurses' contribution to decision making cannot be acknowledged. Much of the background work on which heroic and agentic professional practice rests is carried out by women. In Davies' analysis, nursing

> is not a profession but an adjunct to a gendered concept of profession. Nursing is the activity, in other words, that enables medicine to present itself as masculine/rational and to gain the power and the privilege of doing so.
>
> (1995: 61)

Witz (1992) has analysed the campaign for nurse registration (see Chapter 4) as a campaign for professional autonomy in terms of what Davies (1995) describes as a 'masculinist vision'. The pro-registration campaign looked to the state to grant nurses the autonomy to

> determine the standard and duration of nurse education, to control entry into the ranks of nurses, and to improve their pay and conditions. The core of pro-registrationist nurses' professional project was the demand for 'self-government' and this was posed as an alternative to the 'subjugation' of nurses.
>
> (Witz 1992: 128)

The campaign employed the strategies of usurpation and exclusion. It sought to usurp the power of the hospitals as employers through controlling nurse training and pay and conditions. It sought to limit the power of the medical profession on any controlling statutory body for nursing. In addition, Witz argues, pro-registrationists sought to control nurses' position in the labour market through exclusionary tactics, that is, through advocating one portal of entry into the profession and the control of education by a central body. As already seen in Chapter 4, although the campaign for nurse registration was successful, culminating in the Nurse Registration Act 1919, and although a General Nursing Council was established, the campaign failed to bring nurses autonomous professional status. In attempting to diminish the influence of the hospital over the recruitment of nurses and the conditions of nurses' work, the registration movement could be seen as reducing women's (matrons') power in the organisations, in favour of attempts to increase professional autonomy.

As Witz (1992: 202) notes, nurses' professionalising project resurfaced in the 1980s through the Project 2000 educational reforms. Although these reforms brought supernumerary status to students, abolished the two grades of qualified nurse by ending enrolled nurse training and largely denied support workers the title of 'nurse' by replacing nursing auxiliaries with 'health care assistants', nurse education remains influenced by the health service through health care Trust representatives on education purchasing consortia. Responsibility for the education of nurses rests with higher education institutions, forcing professional bodies to share responsibility for educational standards. While these arrangements may eventually assist nurses to develop more autonomous roles within health care, nursing as a profession remains constrained by health service labour force requirements. Nurses' pay and conditions are not within the professions' control. Sociology can help to identify the importance of looking at nurses as labour as well as professionals, subordinate to, or independent of, doctors (Miers 1999a).

Challenging gendered cultural codes: a new professionalism

Davies (1995) suggests that nursing's project should not be a professionalising one in the masculinist sense but one that challenges the gendered basis of the concept of profession through reformulating the notion of a health care practitioner. The new caring practitioner would be using the strengths of interdependency, adaptability and co-operative, supportive emotional labour, which may be intrinsic to feminine cultural codes. The new practitioner would be:

- neither distant nor involved but *engaged*;
- neither autonomous nor passive/dependent but *interdependent*;

- neither self-orientated nor self-effacing but accepting of an *embodied use of self* as part of the therapeutic encounter;

- neither instrumental nor passive but a *creator of an active community* in which a solution can be negotiated;

- neither the master/possessor of knowledge nor the user of experience but a *reflective user of experience and expertise.*

(Davies 1995: 149–50)

The challenge implicit in Davies' reformulation of the concept of a profession is also a challenge to the masculinist assumptions inherent in the alliance of autonomy, self-orientation and instrumental agency as well as the association of such attributes with power and productivity. It is a challenge to both a masculinist identity project and the knowledge project. Davies recognises that thinking outside or across gendered cultural codes can change our perceptions of roles and activity. It can also change our perceptions of autonomy, dependency and caring. Orbach's (1998 [1978]) description of a mother's restraint on her daughter's desires to be a 'powerful, autonomous, self-directed, energetic and productive human being' (p. 28) as a *rupture* in development, and a loss to be recompensed by taking care of other, places giving to others in opposition to power, autonomy and self-direction. Taking care of other and giving to others are presented as deriving from the daughter's own need for emotional support and growth, and from the restraint on the capacity to be an energetic and productive human being. Other-orientation is presented as a recompense for loss of self-direction. Caring is (perversely) presented as a passive response, not the autonomous action of a productive human being. Caring is seen as deriving from dependency rather than choice. Davies' (1995) concept of a new practitioner helps to unmask gendered assumptions about human agency and care. As already noted, these assumptions are also culturally specific. Western models of rationality and autonomy are not shared world wide.

Interdependence in health care

Davies' concept of a new practitioner can be seen as supportive of the emphasised importance of professionals working in partnership with users and carers to promote health. Health-promoting actions have been characterised as involving holism, equity and collaboration (Cribb and Dines 1993). Macleod Clark (1993) has defined 'health nursing' as involving collaborative individualised, negotiated supportive and facilitative processes. As such, 'health nursing' interactions differ from 'sick-nursing' interactions described as 'nurse dominated, generalised, prescriptive, reassuring and directive' (Latter 1998: 13). Although nurses' emotional labour skills may be seen as deriving from a gendered subordinate and from subservience to medical roles, health promotion literature suggests that such skills may be empowering for the patient or client (Kendall 1998).

It has also been suggested, however, that nurses cannot empower unless they themselves are empowered (Lask 1987, Rodwell 1996, Tones 1998). Latter's report of a study of nurses' health promotion activity in three different wards found that the interaction with clients most closely approximated to a health-promoting approach among nurses on a ward organised on primary nursing principles (Latter 1998). Latter argues that it is the autonomy and control implicit in the philosophy of primary nursing that empowered the nurses to develop their health-promoting potential. Primary nursing as a care philosophy offers primary nurses autonomy from nursing hierarchy and a more autonomous one-to-one relationship with 'their' patients, albeit a collaborative one. Such autonomous practice can be seen as facilitated by nursing's professional body, the United Kingdom Central Council for Nursing, Midwifery and Health Visiting (UKCC), through the publication of the *Scope of Professional Practice* (UKCC 1992), which gave the responsibility for the development of professional roles to individual practitioners, thus fostering an autonomous awareness of individual professional responsibility rather than placing the responsibility for nurses' development with managers.

Primary nursing may be seen as an important development for nursing by those who regard nurses' potential in health care and health promotion as being severely limited by their own subordination as a profession. If nurses' lack of individualised autonomy is seen as a problem, and the achievement of a masculinist notion of professionalism as a solution, primary nursing may be an important way forward. However, despite Latter's findings concerning the relative success of primary nurses in health-promoting interaction and other research showing the effectiveness of primary nursing as a method of organising care (Pearson 1988), primary nursing has been shown to be vulnerable to cost cutting measures and Trust management-initiated reorganisations. Savage (1995) found that the disbanding of a primary nursing ward on which nurses had generated their own ethos and interactive style resulted in personal difficulties for the nurses involved. The achievements of relative autonomy for nurses in a specific setting for a specific period did not lead to significant, lasting, empowerment for individuals or for the profession. Savage notes that once the nurses were unable to practise primary nursing according to their 'visionary ethos', many 'were thrown into professional and personal crisis' (Savage 1995: 120). The pursuit of professional status and autonomy for nurses may not enable nurses to sustain collaborative health nursing. Both nurses and clients are part of health care teams working within organisations. For this reason, Davies' notion of a collaborative, facilitative and interdependent professional rather than autonomous practitioners may be a considerably more realistic and effective model for nursing to adopt. Annandale (1996) found that nurses and midwives do not necessarily welcome increased autonomy. They fear reprisals, such as disciplinary action, for minor errors in a climate in which patients are more aware of their rights.

An analysis of empowerment that takes into account nurses' other-orientation and the potential of nurses' emotional labour may be that of self-efficacy theory (Bandura 1977). Self-efficacy theory suggests that an individual's perceptions of personal efficacy determines whether or not an action is attempted and whether or not an individual perseveres to overcome obstacles and achieve success. For the autonomous practitioner to demonstrate efficacy in health promotion, other-orientation would be essential since health promotional activities using a self-efficacy framework necessitate an individual's 'full involvement and control' (Sturt 1998: 43). The client, rather than the professional is in control. Health promotion practice linked to self-efficacy theory can 'enable the patient to begin to take control of the consultation and the processes and objectives which emerge from it. In this way the individual can engage in the empowering process' (Sturt 1998: 44).

This is not a model of practice that brings power to the professional. On the contrary, it is empowering for the client. From this theoretical model, the professional is an other-orientated, productive human being bringing control to others. If self-efficacy is empowering and nurses' perceptions of efficacy rest in their other-orientated emotional labour (their care), it is clear that nurses do not need to feel powerful in a power-as-autonomy sense in order to empower through health care. Perceptions of self-efficacy as carers may be more important than perceptions of autonomy, power and control. Interdependency does not mean dependency; care does not mean control, or the lack of it. Perceptions of self-efficacy as a carer characterise neither autonomy nor dependence but may involve both. Such perceptions are predicated on engagement and shaped through reflection. Such perceptions are not easily framed through masculine or feminine cultural codes. The difficulties that nurses may have in developing their role as engaged professionals in the interdependent health care team may relate to the gendered nature of the organisations in which they work.

8 Gender and health care management

Introduction

Nurses' role in health care management is constrained by gendered organisational cultures. Chapter 5 has indicated ways in which linking the profession with a restricting discourse of femininity through romanticised and sexualised media imagery in the 1950s and 60s had a constraining effect on nursing's development. The subordination of nursing to the medical profession and the denigratory imagery was accompanied by the post-World War Two diminution of nurses' influence through changes in hospital management structures. The development of the NHS diluted rather than enhanced the nurses' role in the management of the health service.

The matron's declining role in the NHS

Prior to the development of the NHS, matrons were part of the policy making management team of most hospitals and had considerable influence via their control over the 'housekeeping' functions of the hospital – linen rooms, laundries, female domestics and catering staff. Through such control, the matron had 'control over the running of the wards, departments and most services relative to total patient management: she had control over the patient's environment' (White 1985: 59). After nationalisation, the matron's power was reduced in two significant ways: she lost part of her empire to hospital administrators, and she lost her direct access to the policy making mechanism for the hospital – the Hospital Management Committee. These changes could also be placed in a broader context. The matron's role developed through a model of female management over households that was familiar in middle- and upper-class households that depended on 'the lady of the house' supervising a hierarchy of domestic

143

servants. By the time of the development of the NHS, nursing's model of female management was no longer replicated in miniature in domestic settings, and there was no counterpart in the public settings of industry and offices. Models of management in the public world were masculine models.

At the inception of the NHS, 2,835 hospitals with 388,000 beds became its responsibility. Over half the hospitals had fewer than 200 beds; hence the 14 regional hospital boards established to oversee the process grouped hospitals together to be managed by Hospital Management Committees (HMC). The HMC had an administrator called a group secretary. Each individual hospital had a hospital secretary or unit administrator and a matron. Both administrators and matrons had to report to the HMC through the group secretary, thus, in effect, reducing the direct influence of the matron (White 1985). White reports that most matrons did not even receive papers for the management committee meetings (p. 56). Group finance officers and group supplies officers were also members of the HMCs, and there was statutory provision for medical representation on both regional hospital boards and hospital management committees. Doctors established their own medical staff committees at hospital level and advisory groups at group level.

Some management committees set up nursing advisory committees, but, in general, nursing's representation at regional and group level was minimal. White suggests that nurses did not recognise the significance of involvement in policy making at group level, and matrons were reluctant to argue for the establishment of a group matron position because of a reluctance to consider the possibility of conceding their own authority to the matron of another hospital. Insecurity led matrons to fear each other and to act in defence of their own interests rather than in the interests of the profession. Although matrons in teaching hospitals appear to have retained their influence, through continuing to relate directly to the Board of Governors, matrons were placed in a significantly different position after the inception of the NHS from that which they had hitherto occupied. Matrons were still responsible for nursing and for training schools, but, as White points out, 'the administrators had become responsible for the environment in which the nurses had to function' (1985: 60). These changes left the matron with a lack of clarity about her role and function. She found it difficult to play her role as spokeswoman for nurses, lacking direct access to the HMC. She received no training for her new role in a changed system, and 'the questioning of the matron's right to represent her nurses was received as a blasphemy that added further to her insecurity' (White 1985: 65).

Matrons did not react well to these changes. White attributes their defensive anxiety to nurses' carefully cultivated variant of femininity – 'the dependence and pliant credulity of the gentle-woman of the Victorian era' – coupled with their 'political ingen-uousness and social inexperience' (p. 61), characteristics that were embedded in gendered assumptions about femininity at that time. White identifies further difficulties faced by the matrons: nurses' role was changing. The importance of bedside nursing care allowing vigilance through the stages of infectious disease was lessening as effective drug therapies were developed. New drugs and treatment routines, however, meant that new skills were necessary to support medical work.

> The nurses were not prepared for this shift and found that their skills, which had once been acclaimed, were being adversely criticised as unprofitable, repetitive duties which less well-trained staff should take over. Furthermore, the doctors were persistently relegating more technical tasks to nurses who were not trained for them and who felt that, by accepting them, they were neglecting their own duties.

> Another difficulty facing the matrons was the shortage of recruits for nurse training. There was no minimum education requirement for recruits since this had been abandoned in 1939. The HMCs, who relied on student nurses for labour, pressed the matrons to increase their numbers of students. The matrons had no objective criteria for the screening and selection of candidates and relied on their own judgment. The lack of an objective standard made it difficult for the matrons to withstand pressure from their authorities, and their aspirations to maintain 'professional standards' often succumbed to bureaucratic priorities.
>
> (White 1985: 61)

Fifty years later, nurse managers face similar difficulties.

Returning to fifty years ago, matrons began to find themselves losing control of nurse education. The grouping of hospitals through the development of the NHS led to a grouping of nurse training schools. As the schools became larger, a hierarchy developed among nurse tutors, and senior and principal tutors became educationalists, challenging the authority of the matron.

Educationalists began to emphasise the importance of the role of the nurse in individualised patient care, advocating a more student- and patient-centred philosophy that sat uneasily alongside the traditional controlling and supervisory approach of senior nursing staff. Matrons, as general nurses with no further education, lacked the range of skills for their role in a changing NHS. In terms of Weber's (1948) types of authority, they had hitherto been able to draw upon charismatic, traditional and rational-legal authority to maintain their power, but, as models of nursing and of management (as well as of femininity) changed, they were probably less able to rely on charismatic authority or on rational-legal authority, being increasingly forced to rely on tradition as an unsatisfactory source of influence. Not only did their influence decline, but so, too, did their salary. Differentials between the matron's salary and those of lower grades were deliberately held down, and as the matron's salary depended on the number of beds in the hospital, individual salaries were reduced as wartime emergency beds and psychiatric beds were closed. New nursing posts necessary for expanding departments such as theatres or outpatients fitted uneasily into the established nursing grades of staff nurse, sister and assistant matron, leaving nursing seemingly unable to respond flexibly to the needs of a developing health service. It was against this background that the Salmon committee was established to review nurse management structures (MoH and SHDD 1966).

It is easy to be critical of nurse leaders at the time of the creation of the NHS for their lack of understanding of the power politics involved in organisational change in developing the NHS. It is also easy to forget that matrons had few female counterparts in management positions in public services at that time. The role that matrons had performed in hospitals prior to the NHS was little understood by those outside the system. In small hospitals, matrons did not want to lose the control and contact that they had through being able to know the staff personally and personally oversee the patient's environment. The matron's changing administrative role in larger institutions with more complex bureaucratic structures was neither wanted nor well understood. This lack of understanding was, as White (1985) notes, due not so much to a lack of education but to the restrictive nature of a woman's education at that time. Women were not expected to understand the intricacies of political and financial matters. Matrons at the time of the NHS had been trained during the 'lady bountiful' ethos of the voluntary hospitals. White observes:

> So strong was the ideology of the voluntary hospital system and so powerful was the status of the voluntary hospital doctors and nurses that the municipal hospitals, funded from local authority budgets, sought to simulate the same ethos. But this ethos was geared towards the feminine values of caring, sacrifice and subsidiary status. These qualities were not appropriate to the new climate of managerialism and the pursuit of power.
>
> (1985: 84)

Thus, nurses' difficulties in management derived from the dominant constructions of femininity that had shaped the profession. The dominant constructions of masculinity and femininity had also allowed doctors and nurses to work alongside each other in a manner reminiscent of the Victorian 'separate spheres' view of male/female worlds. The system had, however, worked effectively. Into this stable structure came the administrator, with a consequent shift of responsibility and lines of authority. The formal rules did not match the informal relationships, and there was antagonism towards the administrators, who were seen as the agents of change. Highly functional ideologies became attached to social structures as a defence, serving to unify social groups (Sofer 1955).

The ideology attached to the matron was that she represented the interests not only of the nurses, but also of the patients and all female staff. Few matrons could see beyond this defensive ideology. They failed to identify, for example, the need for a voice in the strategic management of the hospital or health service and the importance of acknowledging the need for financial control. The matron defended her position through stern discipline and ritualistic behaviour. Menzies (1970) argued that nurses sought to reduce the burden of responsibility (which can be seen as having increased through changes in policy and in medical practice) by substituting ritualistic behaviour for decision making, redistributing responsibility upwards and engaging in checks and counterchecks to allay anxiety. Thus, the social system inhibited individual nurses' ability to exercise autonomy and make individual decisions. Their 'social system inhibited their capacity for creative or abstract thought and conceptualisation; it interfered with judgment and provoked mistakes' (White 1985: 87). More intelligent recruits were less likely to stay in nursing. The system excluded those who might have been able to explore new ways of enhancing nurses' position.

Organisations and masculinity

Those who did enter nurse management and remained there tended to be men. Female nurses appear to have had difficulty tolerating diversity in models of femininity beyond the already surprisingly divergent stereotypes of angel, sexy nurse, dragon, good woman and lady bountiful. (Political activist, feminist, intellectual and hippie were rare femininities within nursing). The rate of career progression of men within nursing suggests that diverse masculinities have been more easily tolerated. Men's progression, however, could also have been prompted by male nurses' deliberate attempts to move outside and beyond the restrictive discourses of female-dominated staff groups. The Salmon Report recommended a bureaucratic hierarchy of nurse managers, adopting the masculinist notions of management that were dominant at the time (MoH and SHHD 1966).

It is now commonplace to acknowledge the salience of gender in notions of management and organisations (Davies 1995, Collinson and Hearn 1996, Halford *et al*. 1997). Halford *et al*. (1997) identify three alternative approaches to the study of gender and organisations:

1. *contingent*, which sees bureaucracy as gender neutral but male power as deriving from their managerial positions, and from male homosociability;
2. *essentialist,* which sees bureaucracy as a specifically male way of organising, associated with characteristics of the category 'man';
3. *embedded*, which suggests that 'organisational designs, practices and cultures are constructed within economic, social and cultural processes that are always already gendered' (Halford *et al*. 1997: 13).

The embedded approach argues that Weber's own account of rationality, which he saw as being best preserved through bureaucratic structures, has itself an 'unthematised, gendered subtext' that excludes 'the personal, the sexual, and the feminine' from any definition of rationality (Halford *et al.* 1997: 14). It can thus be argued that managerial and organisational logic led the Salmon Report (MoH and SHHD1966) to suggest a bureaucratic system of nursing management. This bureaucratic system was imposed on a social system that was already shaped by gendered constructions of women's (nurses') subordination, dependence and irrationality, and men's (doctors' and administrators') leadership, action and decision making.

Davies (1995) explores the gendering of organisations by first noting the visibility of masculinity in management. It is men who are managers, and hence managerial functions are associated with men; women are in the majority in clerical and administrative roles, and the tasks they perform are hence associated with femininity. The visibility of femininity in many hospital settings (but not necessarily in places for care of the mentally ill) means that it can seem natural that femininity fits women for the 'intricate work' of nursing care. The gendered expectations concerning roles and hierarchies can lead to difficulties for individuals 'who are "out of the ordinary" in terms of the expected sexual division of labour' (Davies 1995: 46). Such individuals have to manage interaction cues with care and make compromises when gender rules appear to conflict with organisational role expectations. Male nurses are aware of this. Halford *et al.* (1997), reporting on their research concerning men and women in health care, note:

> There is a clear onus placed on male nurses to refute the suspicions raised by their presence on the wards by negotiating non-hegemonic and more acceptable forms of masculinity. To this end it appears that male nurses are prepared to carry out considerable 'relational work' and that, in return, female nurses will also work to ease the accommodation of men into ward life.

(p. 237)

Subtleties, or unsubtleties, of gendered interaction styles can play a key part in generating organisational cultures, and it is through organisational cultures that masculinity can be sustained as an organisational norm. The language of management can often be couched in terms of military prowess. There are mission statements, campaigns and price wars, targets, battles and competitors. Management is mastery over self, over others, over objects, through technology and science, over others' labour (Holloway 1996). Organisational cultures can be sexualised and heterosexualised (Pringle 1989, Kanter 1993, Adkins 1995). Gender is also embedded in the abstract logic of an organisation. Drawing on Acker's work (1990), Davies notes the gendered nature of the notions of job hierarchy and career, all of which assume the working life of a male able to participate in the organisation free from the responsibilities of home and family. To sustain the importance of such freedom from concerns outside the organisation, organisations run on an impersonal, rational, instrumental logic that is able to exclude the emotional and practical world that supports the workers' individual and embodied needs. The importance of the literature exploring the gendered nature of management and organisations lies in the recognition that approaches to enhancing opportunities for women that concentrate on ensuring equality of opportunity for women in existing organisational structures are unlikely to be effective if the embedded masculinity of the organisational culture remains.

Men in nursing management

In the 1960s, male progression into nurse management before and after the Salmon Report was probably facilitated by the contingency of changing managerial functions and by dominant assumptions about masculinity and femininity. Lloyd (1965), a male Principal Nursing Officer, argued that men would bring a quality of leadership totally new to nursing. He saw men as being particularly suited for new responsibilities:

> The responsibilities of the principal nursing officer are rather different from those of the chief male nurse and somewhat more exacting. He emerges as the sole nursing representative, given equal status with the medical and lay administrator and with a new image in the field of public relations.

In addition to his responsibilities for staffing, training and nursing standards, he is called upon to give advice in planning both for buildings and methods. He is expected to organise large-scale occupational and rehabilitation programmes for the long-term patient. The male practical mind is invaluable in this sphere and he is able to talk in the same terms as the trades foreman and technician-joiner.

(Lloyd 1965: 363)

Reflecting further on his experiences in management, Lloyd notes that 'it is necessary to take account of the fact that women generally tend to react to most problems and situations in an emotional rather than a rational manner'. His view is that

women are far better at persisting with a set routine. Once a particular nursing policy is decided they can be relied upon to 'stick at it' to the bitter end, no matter what difficulties ensue... male administration is more progressive, dynamic and adventurous than its female counterpart.

(Lloyd 1965: 364)

With the publication of such views in *Nursing Times*, the recruitment of men into management posts in nursing seems almost inevitable. It is interesting to note the author's identification of the importance of 'the male practical mind' as distinct from the female ability to stick to a set routine: women for the mundane; men for progress. Nevertheless, Lloyd notes some female skills. They are 'more loyal than their male counterparts and are also much more ready to accept a temporary compromise' (Lloyd 1965: 364). He records an example of women subordinates taking advantage of his deliberately participative management style by ordering for themselves a supply of the most expensive uniforms. Behind the male/female dichotomous rhetoric, his examples suggest an atmosphere of co-operation and negotiation.

Evans (1997) has argued that it is males in nursing who gain the benefits of female nurses' co-operation. Her view is that the entrance of men into nursing does not mean that masculine and feminine roles are progressively integrated. On the contrary, she argues, male nurses use strategies that distance them from the feminine image of nurses, to their own advantage. She sees men in nursing as illustrating Kanter's concept of tokenism. Tokens are people who differ from the majority by an ascribed characteristic such as race or sex and hence bring with them associated cultural assumptions (Kanter 1977). We have already identified the cultural links between masculinity and management. Evans argues that the ease with which men in nursing are able to take advantage of their masculinity as cultural capital in the world of management is facilitated by nurses' feminine and professional caring ideology (Kauppinen-Toropainen and Lammi 1993, Villeneuve 1994):

> When such an ideology is coupled with the notion that men are valuable, special or unique, the occupational climate that results is characterised by women nurses who consciously or unconsciously support and nurture the careers of men colleagues.
>
> (Evans 1997: 227)

Roberts (1983) has argued that such behaviour on the part of women can be seen as characteristic of oppressed group behaviour. Nurses are an oppressed group who perceive themselves in terms of the oppressor's view of reality and hence perceive themselves as inferior. Female nurses accept a masculinist view of management that excludes themselves but not their male colleagues. Such an analysis may well oversimplify the motivations of individual nurses, but a non-oppressed, femininist, view of management skills would enhance nurses' awareness of the managerial importance of their own nurturing and supportive skills. Paradoxically, men in nursing who receive facilitative support from women colleagues, which enhances their career, may well learn from such support, helping them to develop their own facilitative managerial skills, albeit skills that may not feature strongly in the masculinist management imagery.

Compatibility with cultural constructions of masculinity may also help to explain the presence of male nurses in 'islands of masculinity' (Egeland and Brown 1988) within the profession. These include:

> psychiatry because of its association with physical strength; anaesthesiology, because of its association with technical prowess and autonomy; and, intensive and emergency care, because of their association with technical prowess and cool-headedness.
>
> (Evans 1997: 226)

Further factors that advantage men in the profession are 'breadwinner' roles within family structures and higher educational qualifications. Williams (1989) found that married women nurses are less likely than single women to pursue advanced degrees and that men applying for promotion have higher qualifications than women. Evans concludes that men in nursing will not change the gendered nature of the profession as long as male nurses see it as being to their advantage to separate themselves from the most 'feminine' areas of nursing in order to support their own masculinity. Ratcliffe (1996), however, presents a more sophisticated analysis of the rise of men in nursing management, identifying the role of geographical mobility in the job market as a type of closure against women who, for family reasons, are not able to move. In a market that values experience from outside, lack of opportunities for geographical mobility serve as barriers to promotion.

Despite a concern that the presence of men in nursing management and in nursing itself has had little effect on the gendered and limiting nature of assumptions about the profession, there has been little research into the difference, if any, between men's and women's management styles in health care. Valentine (1995) has reviewed research into gender differences in the management of conflict and identified that the majority of studies show that women use compromising as a management style more often than men. Avoiding was also a style of conflict management adopted by women. In Valentine's (1988) case study in a Canadian hospital school of nursing, she found that nurse educators' major method of managing conflict was avoidance. American studies also identified avoidance as the most frequent approach to conflict management adopted by staff nurses, nurse managers relying on compromise. In general, competition was the strategy used least often, collaborating and accommodating being used less frequently than avoidance or compromise and more frequently than competition.

In further reviews of explanations for nurses' use of compromise and avoidance as management styles in the face of conflict, Valentine notes the associations with women's socialisation into meeting others' needs, dilemmas over expressions of conflict that may seem to contradict caring and supportive ideologies, and the view that compromise is a frequently used response in situations of power differentials (Johnson 1994). Although expressing concern that avoidance and compromise may not be the most effective management styles, Valentine notes that organisational theories explaining men's behaviour may not necessarily explain women's behaviour. A further exploration of women's management styles would be helpful in trying to understand both nurses' role in management and future patterns for management in health care. With the current emphasis on interprofessional working, co-operation, participation and equity in the new NHS (DoH 1997), collaboration is being acknowledged as preferable to competition. However, the avoidance of conflict may be an unhelpful management style.

Gilloran (1995), in a study of differences between male and female care delivery and supervisory styles in psychogeriatric nursing, found that male and female nurses had some stereotypical views about each others' abilities and approaches. Females saw men as being reluctant to get involved in 'heavy' nursing care. Females saw themselves as being more organised, tidy and attentive to detail in caring for clients. Men saw themselves as more able to take decisions. Women saw men as being more concerned with the paperwork, office work and relatives, reflecting different priorities. The benefits of a mixed gender staff team were appreciated by all, both men and women perceiving the value of different perspectives. The presence of men acting to ameliorate female 'bitchiness' was noted by both sexes. When asked about men and women in supervision, males were seen as being more rational and academic in their approach, while women were seen as more approachable (Gilloran 1995). The benefits of combining these attributes seem obvious for nursing, as in other areas of work.

Women's more accessible management styles have been noted in other professions (Grimwood and Popplestone 1993, Ozga 1993). Grimwood and Popplestone list the eight areas in which Loden (1985) identified women as managing differently from men:

1. Women use power differently, focusing on empowering rather than personal power acquisition.
2. Women problem solve using 'intuitive' and 'rational' information.
3. Women use a wide range of interpersonal skills.
4. Women tend to be team focused, using team skills.
5. Women are concerned with standard setting and take risks to improve quality.

6. Women focus on managing diversity, stress and boundaries but are more successful in helping others to develop such skills than themselves.
7. Women seek win–win solutions to handling conflict.
8. Women pitch in if necessary and value professional development for all.

This approach challenges hierarchical management structures. Many of these descriptions of women's approaches could – and probably do – describe a desirable management style for males or females managing nursing teams.

'New wave' management

Increasingly, it is a 'feminine' style of management that is advocated as part of a 'new wave' of management practices. The origins of such practices may lie in post-Fordist approaches to the efficient use of labour, relying on 'core' and 'periphery' workers to provide the most flexible organisational form, best able to cope with increased competition (Atkinson 1986). In service industries and personal service professions, flexibility is needed to respond to the changing needs of the clients and, in the NHS, the increased emphasis on client participation in decision making and improving the quality of the client's experience (DoH 1989b). A responsiveness to clients in all service and manufacturing sectors demands high levels of social skill among employees, introducing a new emphasis on interpersonal skills at all levels of the organisa-tion. Flexible organisations have introduced flatter, horizontal structures, reliant on teamwork and peer networks, arguably cemented by shared and individual responsibility and autonomy in the name of participation and empowerment.

New methods of management call for new forms of human engagement 'wherein the role of social relationships is paramount' (Kerfoot and Knights 1996: 95). Since the social relationships take place in situations in which there is an absence of clear lines of instrumental control, those accustomed to masculinist models of management can feel particularly uncomfortable. To make new forms of management work, as Goleman (1998) argues, closer attention has to be paid to what he terms 'emotional intelligence', that is, the management of one's own and others' feelings. As Kerfoot and Knights (1996) note, the danger is that if masculinist management appropriates the new concern for developing skills in teamwork, emotional intelligence and human relations, for purely instrumentalist purposes, the humanising purpose of managerial cultural change will be lost. Such cultural change is only likely if it is part of a deeper cultural shift in the construction of masculinities and femininities.

Such a change may be possible. Health care could be an appropriate site of cultural change. The new management philosophies, although predicated on an analysis of successful business survival strategies, promote the discourses of participative health care. Perry (1993) claims that

> companies which survive and thrive in the modern economy are those which achieve devolved decision-making, where people feel they have control over the day-to-day conditions of their working lives; where central management is an enabler rather than a controller; a setter of frameworks and a creator of environment and tone, rather than a conventional arbiter of staff fortunes.

(pp. 92–3)

Interestingly, Pauline Perry (1993), the first female vice-chancellor of a polytechnic, in describing her own route to senior educational management, identified the formative managerial skills she had learned while at home caring for her young family. These she describes as nurturance, trust and patience, listening skills, taking feelings into account, releasing control, and enabling leadership. Her account is important since she is identifying how she drew upon her experiences in her conventionally expected role as a mother – a good woman – as a basis for understanding managerial roles in education.

In nursing, a century earlier, 'good women' drew similarly on their experience in managing a household to develop careers in nursing. However, the 'lady bountiful' nurses of Victorian times were not as well placed as educated mothers in the 1950s and 60s to develop and apply their enabling and nurturing skills to their profession. The 'lady bountiful' leaders of nursing were accustomed to a Victorian hierarchical and repressive patriarchal management style, which they applied in a protective manner to the nurses and patients for whom they were responsible. Despite the differences in types of domestic preparation for management roles, however, it is probable that the matrons of the past used compromise and co-operation to manage conflict and tensions.

In the masculinist management eras that have predominated since the development of scientific management (Taylor 1947) and been exacerbated through the competitive rhetoric of market philosophies, women's co-operative management skills may have been devalued, leading to the defensive adoption of avoidance as a method of managing conflict and a reluctance to accept responsibilities for decision making.

The extent to which management philosophies may now be changing can, however, be overemphasised. In addition, the management of the health service is, in the interests of the public, always subjected to control by the state and regulatory professional bodies. The possibilities of external monitoring through the Commission for Health Improvement and the National Institute for Clinical Excellence may prompt further changes in management practices (DoH 1997).

Organising the organisation: gender and practice

Embedded in the discussion so far are additional gendered assumptions about management that have received very little attention in the literature. We have already noted Lloyd's (1965) distinction between the male 'practical mind' and female perseverance with routine. This is easily seen as a distinction between the active decision maker and the subservient follower of rules. Gilloran (1995) noted similar gendered differences in self-perception between male and female nurses. Women see themselves as attentive to detail; men see themselves as decision makers. Men's action is disembodied; they take strategic decisions. Women's action is embodied; they get things done, through an observant, constant attentiveness to the detail ensuring that the organisation is organised – not just the practical mind but the practical activity. Like emotional labour, such practical activity (filing, tea making or checking observations) can be presented as occurring without the benefit of thought, even the thought of the practical mind.

Women's activities are perceived as being independent of the strategic overall aim of the organisation. Filing, tea making and checking observations can be denigrated as being routinised, ignoring their possible strategic role in, for example, patient care. Male actions, however reactive and habitual, are the sign of the agentic strategist. Female actions are unimportant and taken for granted. Organisations may be gendered male, yet it is women who are perceived as good at organising.

Organising, unlike managing an organisation, is often seen as a feminine skill, probably because of the implicit involvement of social skills. Organising involves communicating with others to ensure that actions are co-ordinated. Organising unites being and doing, strategy and detail, and brings organic living unity to a structure. Nursing is an organising as well as a caring activity, as the matrons understood. If their manner of hierarchical control became outdated, it has not removed the importance of co-ordinating the activities that contribute to a safe environment for promoting health. James recognises the importance of nursing as an organising activity in her writings on care, work and organisation. She recognises that is not just emotional labour that is involved in care:

> emotional labour also needs a form of organisation and management different to the rigidity of the work ethic where principles of predictability and control dominate. 'Care' as emotional labour requires the flexibility to respond to different circumstances as they arise in ways that cannot be strictly timetabled, but nevertheless, have an internally coherent form of organisation.
>
> (1992b: 106)

The principles involved in 'care' and the labour involved in nursing 'work' are pragmatically aligned in 'carework'. James (1992b) argues that retaining the distinction between 'care' and 'work', as thesis and antithesis, allows the gaps between ideals and practice to be noticed. Aligning them in a pragmatic synthesis as 'carework' highlights, in addition, the importance of nurses' organising activities within health care and in the workplace.

PART IV

Caring for men, caring for women

---

9   Gender-sensitive care

Introduction

This chapter argues that understanding gender as a cultural construction has the potential to improve the quality of nursing care. Gender-sensitive care depends on a knowledge of the social processes that affect health and illness as well as the social processes affecting the practice of care. Care as an activity and nurses as professionals involved in care are closely associated with women and with cultural codes of femininity. Many of the organisations in which nurses work, however, are shaped by cultural codes of masculinity, particularly through the dominant profession in health care – medicine. Even in community settings and in private homes, nurses and their clients are affected by the influence of gender on work and domestic lives and on health and illness. Earlier parts of this book have looked more closely at gendered cultural codes by identifying masculinities and femininities that have influenced nursing and affect mortality and morbidity. This part attempts to explore the possibilities for gender-sensitive nursing care by reflecting on gendered cultural codes and on different explanatory approaches.

Theoretical approaches

Sharp (1994) has argued that sociological theories are of little use to nurses in their practice. The problem with different theories is that they suggest different guidelines for action. Functionalism, for example, has suggested that the expectations and obligations of men and women are shaped by the social roles that men and women occupy in domestic and work settings. Functionalism was a popular approach in the 1950s and 60s, at a time when divorce was uncommon, men were the breadwinners and women were the family nurturers. Changes in the employment opportunities and in domestic living arrangements expose the limitations of sex-role theory but do not negate the relevance of the view that it might be functional for gender expectations to 'fit' the variety of social roles taken by men and women in any particular social structure. A functionalist approach does not necessarily, of itself, inhibit gender-sensitive care, but rigid adherence to the view that men are the decision makers and providers, and women the home makers and nurturers can bring psychological distress for both men and women. Such rigid views can result in inappropriate care. The challenge for nurses is to understand the way in which deeply embedded assumptions about men's and women's roles permeate professional cultures as well as the cultures of their clients, and to use that understanding to enhance their own practice.

It could be argued that using any nursing model as a basis for planning care will prompt a nurse to consider the effect of work and family roles on the health status of a client. Nursing models encourage a holistic approach to care. Using a nursing model, however, does not necessarily lead to a critical reflection on gendered assumptions and the gendered presentation of self, although male nurses' contravention of male gender expectations may facilitate reflection on notions of masculinity (Clark 1997, MacDougall 1997, Piper 1997). Feminist sociologists have been critical of nurses' sensitivity to the needs of women. Abbott and Wallace (1997) claim that although the paid health care providers are themselves often women, 'they fail to identify with the unpaid carers and assume that women are ready, willing and able to provide the constant care demanded of them' (p. 162). The dominant medical profession has been criticised for acting as a form of patriarchal control over women, using medical knowledge to reinforce women's dependency. 'The giving of tranquillisers to housewives with depression only renders the intolerable more tolerable; it does nothing to alleviate the underlying causes of depression' (Abbott and Wallace 1997: 164).

Nursing research suggests that nurses may demonstrate gender bias in care delivery. Greipp (1996), in an American study of predicted self and colleague reactions to simulated clients found that female nurses demonstrated most favourable reactions to young male clients exhibiting characteristics such as co-operativeness, honesty, compliance and friendliness. Least favourable reactions from the 268 study respondents were towards old, male clients who behaved aggressively, were unco-operative or were demanding. Female nurses do not necessarily enjoy caring for women. Mackay (1989) found that half the student nurses interviewed preferred to nurse males; only three reported a preference for caring for female patients. The students' view was that women complained more than men. Men were seen as more willing to do things for themselves and hence more helpful. Smith (1992) found similar views among student nurses in her study, although nurses found women easier to talk to (Smith 1992).

Both Smith and Mackay observe that not only did the student nurses show an awareness of the social roles that men and women play and the possible effects of these roles on their behaviour in the public setting of the hospital, but also the students' own expectations of male and female roles could affect their care. Women tended to be seen as taking advantage of their stay in hospital by relinquishing their normal (extensive) domestic responsibilities. Men, on the other hand, were seen as preferring to maintain a public appearance of independence. Smith notes that the nurses 'resented having to do things for female patients which the patients, as women, usually did for others. They were harder on the women because of this, and expected more gratitude from them' (Smith 1992: 62).

Both the data and the analyses presented here warrant caution, however. Greipp's study relied on simulated clients and on a low response rate. Studies of nurses' patient preferences are limited, and the youth and inexperience of students cast doubt on the relevance of the Mackay's and Smith's data. Nevertheless, such comments confirm that female nurses have not necessarily been sensitive to women's care needs and demonstrate the importance of considering our own assumptions about gender and gender roles and their effect on our work and relationships.

Gender is a relational concept; gender constructions develop through relationships. Nursing is a relationship. Nurses and clients respond to the way in which others respond to them. In my own observations recorded as a student nurse, I noted the lack of rapport between women nurses and other professional women:

> I must note the interprofessional rivalries and labelling that goes on especially between women. Women teachers and social workers on our ward present a hostile face to nurses, they clearly don't want to trust them and

to treat them well and so they don't 'give' to nurses in any way – no rewards, no thanks. And nurses resent... what?... their higher professional status? easier job? more pay? their assumed superiority? or simply their detached and distant attitude, lack of friendliness? And so nurses devalue them: 'if that's what teachers/social workers are like no wonder we're in a mess'.

(Miers, notes as a student nurse 6/3/87)

Although my own observations suggest that professional status divisions may inhibit gender-sensitive nursing care, Brooks and Phillips (1996), from a postal questionnaire study of women's primary health care needs and perceptions of care, found that many women valued 'the lack of social distance in their relationship with nurses' (p. 1210). However, younger women were less positive about their experience of care from a practice nurse than were women over 40.

Feminisms and gender-sensitive care

In 1987, as a mature student nurse with varied work experience as a social scientist, I was curious to know whether feminism might provide a supportive standpoint for gender-sensitive health care. My view of feminism, at that time, was that it had successfully highlighted the pervasive power of patriarchy and the consequent denigration of my concurrent roles as mother and student nurse, but had neither highlighted the intricacies and the skill involved in those roles nor alleviated the denigration. As a student, I tried to record what I learnt about nursing:

I learn that motherhood and domestic demands are too similar to nursing – women get no release/reprieve. I learn that it is possible to wash patients in ways that make them feel like a lump of meat. I learn that when speed is a priority, nursing isn't. Yet although I don't like what I see, I don't lose respect for the nurses who work like that. Their petty concerns about their own status arise because the world gives them so little to be thankful for.

(Miers, notes as a student nurse, 16/5/87)

Feminism can, however, help to identify the processes that can make nursing appear such a thankless job. Feminisms may help nurses to recognise women's shared concerns and thus aid nurses in meeting women's health care needs. Some nurse educators have argued for the incorporation of feminism into the nursing curriculum. Hagell (1989) argues that feminist theory in nursing could help to 'rekindle the lost emphasis on caring' and illuminate power relationships. Ashley (1980) emphasised the importance of women nurses' status as women and argued strongly that nursing would not become self-directing or effective without 'embracing feminism and all it stands for'. Keddy (1995), however, found that older nurses on post-qualifying courses were initially resistant to a research methodology course that adopted a critical feminist perspective. Nevertheless, they moved quickly from resistance to anger. Keddy adopted a 'shared governance' approach to learning in which course participants and lecturer worked together in non-hierarchical relationships, valuing subjectivity, flexibility and diversity. Students were given time to complete a journal at the end of every session, which Keddy read and responded to regularly. Keddy records a quote from one student's journal:

> I can't get enough of reading about how oppressed I have been all these years. For once my life is starting to make sense. Why haven't I heard more about feminist analysis and research before this? What is wrong with nursing that it has taken so long?
>
> (1995: 693)

As a teacher, Keddy worked with students to move beyond anger towards hope through identifying ways in which their changed views about 'issues of women's health, violence against women, children and elderly people' could, if shared by other nurses, have a significant impact on change.

Heinrich and Witt (1993) consider that feminist approaches can energise nurse education through introducing a paradigmatic shift that values both objective and subjective knowledge. It links abstract theory with subjective experience: 'learning became exciting when personal experience was enlightened by theoretical understanding' (p. 118). Heinrich and Witt drew on Wheeler and Chinn's (1991) emphasis on praxis, that is, the interconnection between values and action. The shared self-disclosure facilitated through feminist approaches to education becomes, Wheeler and Chinn argue, a way of enabling the power of nurturing. British literature, however, has been less articulate about incorporating feminism into nurse education, although social science teachers have played their part in ensuring that feminism has a curriculum place.

Allan (1993) has explored the concept of feminism in order to enable her to use feminism to enhance nursing practice and to develop a feminist theory of nursing. She identifies two significant strands in feminist literature: a concern with male domination and a concern with expressing an awareness of oppression through valuing the feminine. Feminist nursing theory or practice could have three empirical referents: a concern with gender equality and equal rights; a concern expressed through theory and action; and valuing individuals for personal qualities rather than biological attributes.

These concerns are echoed in Dominelli's (1997) identification of principles of feminist sociological social work, which she sees as being concerned with understanding status and power relations and their associations with masculinity, identifying processes of exclusion from citizenship and valuing individual experience. Dominelli also specifically identifies the importance of understanding the gendered nature of organisational structures, paid and domestic labour, the welfare state and professionalism.

Whether or not feminism can serve as a basis for nursing theory or for the development of nursing practice depends on views about the nature of knowledge and the relationship between theory and practice. Understanding feminist approaches to nursing research may, therefore, be a necessary prerequisite for a feminist theory of nursing practice. Campbell and Bunting (1991: 7) argue that a feminist epistemology includes the claim that:

- women's experience can be a legitimate source of knowledge – women can be knowers;
- subjective data are valid;
- informants are 'experts' on their own lives;
- knowledge is relational and contextual;
- definitive boundaries between personal and public or personal and political spheres are artificial, as are sharp distinctions between theory and practice.

Such epistemological assumptions lead to research approaches that are based on women's experiences, asking questions that women themselves wish to be addressed in a non-hierarchical relationship between researcher and research participants. Interpretations of the data are shared with the participants, so that participants may benefit. Although there has been lengthy debate in sociological literature about the distinctiveness (or otherwise) of feminist research approaches (Stanley 1990, Hammersley 1992, Ramazonoglu 1992, Oakley 1998), many of the principles of ensuring that research is conducted in an egalitarian, anti-oppressive manner can be seen as exemplifying good practice in health service research and in the practice of health care. Listening to individual experiences and subjective meanings is important in all nursing work. Critics of a distinctive feminist methodology, however, argue that the emphasis on women's own experience is not distinct to feminism but a feature of phenomenological approaches, that all health care research should be critically reviewed for medical (male) bias and that it is almost impossible to study women alone.

Webb (1986) adopted a feminist approach to her research concerning the information needs of women having a hysterectomy. She explains how she moved from a methodological approach involving a researcher asking questions, to an approach in which she shared her own experiences as a gynaecology patient through sharing information with the research participants and listening to their own questions. In this way, the research could answer the questions that the participants wanted answered, and the researcher became involved in supporting the women through making suggestions about their care. Webb's (1986) edited collection on feminist practice in women's health care remains an important contribution to the literature on gender and health care. The contributors identify the principles from which they work. Their shared principles include:

- sharing resources, particularly information, with those with whom they work, thus facilitating informed choice;
- an affirmation of equality, involving sharing power with colleagues and clients;
- facilitating the recognition that problems are not unique to individuals but are shared outcomes of the nature of the society in which we live;
- facilitating mutual support among colleagues and clients.

Webb (1986) identifies nurses' own needs for education to enable them to provide appropriate support for women on gynaecological wards (Webb and Wilson Barnett 1983). On the basis of her research, Webb was able to identify ways in which nurses could enhance their care. These included providing detailed information for women about 'how their bodies work, and how they can expect treatments to affect their physical and emotional health, their family and working lives' (Webb 1986: 109). A knowledge of anatomical and technical terms enables women to ask medical staff for further information, which nurses can further facilitate through initiating discussions in the doctor's presence. Providing written information, talking to family and friends, and bringing women together to share experiences are all activities that nurses could give attention to in providing support for women in their care.

Mary Twomey's account of a feminist approach to district nursing confirms the inadequacy of clients' knowledge about relevant anatomy and physiology. Such knowledge helps to make sense of clients' treatment and allows them to feel involved in their own care and to ask their own questions:

> On several occasions I have visited women who have had a hysterectomy and found that they did not know whether or not they had had their ovaries removed as well – a vital piece of information for most women. The fact that these women do not know whether they have had their ovaries removed reflects their lack of involvement in decision-making about their bodies.
>
> (Twomey 1986: 57)

Mavis Kirkham (1986) discusses midwifery from a feminist perspective. She identifies the importance of listening to women and encouraging them to listen 'to their own bodies and their babies' (p. 37). Kirkham records the relevance of detailed observations of self and client, noting that 'feminist care in labour is grounded in minute observation of the labouring women's reaction' (p. 42):

> In trying different ways of making a woman feel comfortable we state our priorities, and she will be free to tell us when she feels uncomfortable. If we tell her what is happening, she will feel free to tell us her worries. If we give her a running commentary on our actions, we give information.

If we say what we are about to do just before we do it, we give her the opportunity to say 'yes' or 'no' or to make choices without having an exhausting discussion... As well as being aware of the cues we give out, we must be very aware of the cues a woman in labour gives to us. Does her fist pressed into her hip suggest back pain which may be helped by massage, movement or epidural anaesthesia? Does the tightly closed mouth show muscular tension inhibiting the opening of the cervix? If so, how can we best get her to smile?

(Kirkham 1986: 42)

But Kirkham also notes the importance of understanding the organisational context in which care takes place and argues that midwives must also work to improve the system, but not in a way that hurts the women it serves. The bodies of individual women should not be the sites on which confrontations between doctors and midwives are acted out. In contrast to Kirkham's optimism about midwives' ability to make use of detailed observations of self and client, Fleming notes the difficulties of incorporating women's knowledge into documentation. She argues,

It remains the written documentation which is seen by the power holders as 'legitimate'... yet by its very nature midwifery knowledge does not lend itself to documentation. Documentation of midwifery practice for the purposes of client record keeping and audits of practice are therefore carried out in stereotypical form, differing little from records of medical practitioners.

(1998: 13)

Eisner and Wright (1986), in reviewing the possibilities of feminist approaches as general practitioners, discuss the many contradictions of their position as white, privileged female authoritative professionals trying to work with women in an egalitarian and 'sisterly' style that uses to women's advantage, but does not deny, their authority. They found they could use 'doctor's orders' to encourage women to rest and ask for help. In trying to minimise the barriers that derive from their authority as doctors, they acknowledge that they make themselves vulnerable through 'taking on board all the deep distress we encounter every day' (p. 133). Self-revelation helped woman-as-doctor and woman-as-patient to identify together factors that made it difficult for women to change that unhealthy behaviour. Such close, sharing relationships can, however, also risk creating dependency or alternatively a sense of inferiority on the part of clients. Sharing experience, as single mothers for example, may lead to unhelpful comparisons about how women manage their lives. As general practitioners, Eisner and Wright know that they have privileged access to knowledge about the pressures of women's lives and the way in which women undervalue their achievements. 'To help a woman find more purpose for herself' (p. 140) is sometimes possible even in a short consultation.

Eisner and Wright also identify ways in which the insights of feminism can help care for male patients through encouraging a more woman-centred view of the world and allowing men as well as women to question conventional assumptions about male and female roles. One man, made redundant, felt that the main source of his depression was his guilt at being unable to support his wife 'as he was brought up to do'. These authors note that, as professionals, they are often 'unable to avoid reinforcing sex roles which tend to become more rigid under stress such as physical illness when it may not seem an appropriate time to challenge them' (p. 142).

The strengths and weaknesses of a feminist approach to gender-sensitive care may rest in assumptions about the reality of women's shared concerns. Early feminist approaches have been robustly criticised for failing to analyse the complexity and diversity of women's experience and thus simplistically claiming a uniformity of women's standpoint (hooks 1991). Disabled women, for example, have criticised the feminist emphasis on women's right to make their own reproductive decisions (Morris 1993). Nevertheless, the search for uniformity among women can lead to an identification of the principles to be upheld at a policy level that could support the health of all women. As Doyal (1987, 1995) argues, the involvement of women in health policy making is important.

Working as a nurse researcher on a longitudinal study of breast clinic attenders, I recognised the limitations of my own middle-class experience in professional roles and in childcare as a basis for sharing experiences with women. It was the strength of South Wales women and the way in which their caring roles were deeply implicated in that strength that raised my interest in a search for approaches to gender-sensitive care that could appropriately validate women's own experiences, skills and activities.

The unpredictable consequences of physical illness, such as breast cancer can, however, challenge the assumption that sharing experiences is supportive. Encouraging women to share experiences of breast cancer opens women to the unexpected and unwelcome pain of other women's deaths. As Tait notes,

> R's despair because someone else had died was perfectly understandable. The meaning of her breast cancer was dependent on her shared experience with others and her definition of their situation.
>
> (1990: 185)

Support from other women with breast cancer also risks the recognition that other women have different treatment, without necessarily understanding the reasons why this might be the case. Hence sharing experiences complicates and changes the professional's role in support. Tait wrote of her own distress at knowing, but being unable to find satisfactory ways of explaining, that women were treated differently because of the demands of the development of medical knowledge through controlled trials:

> I can remember the acute discomfort of having to work within the hierarchical constraints of the organisation from which I came. It was hard enough to know R's suffering, it was worse to toe the party line and mislead her about the research that was going on.
>
> (p. 186)

The current legal, public and professional emphasis on informed consent to clinical trials should mean that breast care nurses and women with breast cancer no longer suffer such discomfort, but the complexity of the egalitarian sharing of knowledge in disease with uncertain prognosis challenges any practitioner or individual sufferer.

Feminist mental health workers, however, are successfully using their own experiences of powerlessness and oppression to make connections with other women and thereby develop feminist clinical theory and practice (Burstow 1992, Williams and Watson 1996). Holland (1996) describes an innovative model of psychotherapeutic work with depressed women in their own community setting, using a model of mental health intervention that confronts psychological symptoms of depression and social oppression. The use of the model involved four steps in social action psychotherapy which progressed from medical dependency (step one: patients on pills) to taking collective action to demand changes in schools, health centres, community centres, housing and transport (step four: taking action). The intervening stages were step two: person-to-person psychotherapy, in which talking to a woman therapist helped to explore the meanings of depression; and step three: talking in groups, which involved women, together in groups, discovering a common history (HERSTORY) of abuse, misuse and exploitation (Holland 1996).

The model of psychotherapeutic work is a reflexive model of teaching and practice that assumes that therapeutic relationships are more successful if practitioners and clients share analytical approaches. Practitioners who are comfortable with an analytical approach that advocates, for example, desensitising to ameliorate agoraphobia will be more successful with clients who share such a mechanistic view of themselves in the world. Practitioners wishing to challenge oppression will be more successful with assertive and angry service users (Holland 1996). Those with a functionalist analysis of gender roles will work more successfully with clients who do not wish to challenge their sex-identity role. Practitioners adopting a feminist standpoint will enable those already aware of the distress caused by gender constraints. Health care workers with a range of analytical awareness may have the flexibility for effective and varied care that remains gender sensitive.

Men's health and masculinities

Cameron and Bernardes (1998) suggest that the growing literature on masculinity has the potential to help our understanding of health and illness. They particularly welcome the idea that although there is a hegemonic masculinity, there are also multiple masculinities (Connell 1987), and the idea of negotiated gender (Cornwall and Lindisfarne 1994). Hegemonic masculinity can be dangerous to men's health as 'a risk factor in disease aetiology but also a definite barrier to developing a consciousness about health and illness' (Cameron and Bernardes 1998: 128–9). Chronic illness could lead to some men being placed in a position of 'marginalised masculinity' in the gender order (Connell 1987), but for many men, masculinity could be successfully redefined.

Sabo and Gordon (1995) identify how the study of men's health has drawn on the strengths of the work of sex-role theorists and of feminists, and on sociological approaches to inequalities, while avoiding their limitations. Sex-role socialisation theory underestimates the extent to which female domination is reproduced through gender socialisation. Feminist approaches initially overestimated the extent to which women share experiences and underestimated the extent to which hegemonic masculinities lead to structural inequalities between men as well as between men and women. Hegemonic masculinity (emphasising aggressiveness, striving for dominance, competition, size, physical strength and phallocentrism) marginalises different masculinities and constructs a hegemonic femininity (emphasising passivity, physical frailty, a dependence on men, nurturance, co-operation and sexual submissiveness), which 'helps men collectively to maintain their control and domination of women' (Sabo and Gordon 1995: 18). Recognising diversity between men encourages the analysis of aspects of masculinities that can be either health enhancing or health destroying, and under what conditions. An emphasis on physical strength and on control and dominance can help men to work to preserve their health, but aggressiveness, competition and phallocentrism can promote risk taking behaviour that damages the self and others. Femininities also ally with health-enhancing behaviour such as physical cautiousness, risk aversion and stress-reducing nurturance and co-operation, but femininities may also promote passivity (congruent with the sick role) and sexual submissiveness, which can damage women's health.

Many of the principles of feminist praxis can be adopted for the support of men. The Prostate Health Research Project, for example, identified a greater than expected willingness among men to tell their stories and identified substantial unmet need (Cameron and Bernardes 1998). When the organiser of the Prostate Help Association appeared on radio's Jimmy Young Show in 1993, there were thousands of responses, indicating men's need for opportunities to share their experiences about health problems. Nevertheless, they wished to share experiences at a distance: attempts to organise group meetings were unsuccessful. The research project's findings showed how aspects of masculinity, such as the tendency to 'soldier on' and the emphasis on being in control and taking charge, could be seen as resources enabling men to carry on with life despite their chronic health difficulties. Men's individualistic and mechanistic (as opposed to holistic) view of health sometimes led to a detailed monitoring and record keeping of their fluid intake and urinary output, possibly building an individual picture of their condition that allowed them to manage their daily routines successfully.

Some men found, however, that their doctors did not welcome their own 'lay expertise' about their condition. Their detailed knowledge of their symptoms was ignored, and they felt let down by the medical profession. Many men in the study, however, had delayed seeking advice. A 60-year-old man had had symptoms for seven years without consulting health professionals. He noted, 'I lived with it, adapted to the symptoms, didn't define myself as unwell, just accepted it' (Cameron and Bernardes 1998: 124).

Similar ideas concerning caring for men have already been addressed at in the nursing press. Libby Purves (1997), writing in *Nursing Standard,* argues that a 'laddish attitude to health has its plus points as well as its dangers' (p. 19). She notes,

> men do not make friends with illness... If they decide that their health needs attention they either take to violent, life threatening exercise or demand a pill to make them healthier and more virile than ever before. If they have a disease they want it to be definite, so they can square up to it and win.

> (1997: 19)

Piper (1997) also suggests that the cultural construction of masculinity needs to be taken into account when seeking to change men's behaviour that may be damaging their health. Well men's clinics may require men to be passive, submissive and compliant, traits that are contrary to cultural expectations for male behaviour. Piper advocates a self-empowerment approach that 'focuses on the individual's capacity to direct or control his or her own life while acknowledging the wider factors which shape it' (p. 49). Hence the aim should be to encourage men to control their own risk taking behaviour at the same time as working to change patriarchal and socio-economic processes that are destructive to men's health.

Masculinity and nursing

MacDougall (1997), an HIV/palliative care co-ordinator, has explored the concept of masculinity and its relevance to nursing. He looks at the range of approaches to exploring masculinities that have developed over recent years, including the mythopoetic movement initiated by Robert Bly, which sees masculinity as deriving from unconscious patterns, revealed through myths and stories. MacDougall also notes the growth of a men's rights movement, exemplified through the campaign against the Child Support Agency, which united men from different backgrounds. MacDougall examines the significance of the increase in the number of men entering caring professions but suggests that many men in nursing are following traditional masculine patterns in employment by moving into management or working in high-tech areas, carving, as Williams (1989) argues, a 'niche' that allows men to maintain 'masculinity within a feminine context' (1989: 120).

However, gay men, MacDougall suggests, do not follow traditional masculine paths; their experience of being different in the world of dominant masculinities leads to a self-perception that Sullivan suggests is 'more wary and distant, more attuned to appearance and its foibles, more self-conscious and perhaps more reflective' (1995: 198). This sense of marginality in the gender order would be enhanced in a predominantly female profession such as nursing and might further foster a reflectiveness that could promote a sensitivity to others' needs. Alternatively, however, MacDougall notes the danger that the domination of traditional masculinities, underpinned by homophobia, could lead to negative responses by gay men to their own feelings of disempowerment. Disempowered gay men seeking to regain control could resort to negative responses such as racism or sexism, which would reinforce dominant and controlling masculine methods of management. For this reason, MacDougall is sceptical about the potential of male nurses to contribute to changing constructions of masculinity through their own caring behaviour. On the contrary, male nurses could confirm the dominance of a masculine, hierarchical management culture within health care.

Nolan's small study of mental health nurses who had been prisoners of war suggests that the ex-servicemen's model of masculinity has had a longlasting and negative effect on the mental health service. One study respondent said:

> I felt all mixed up after the war. I had a lot of anger and hatred in me at the time. When the bad feelings about the war would come back to me, invariably I would take it out on the patients, and there were even times when I held them responsible for what I had been through. I must have made their lives hell. Looking back, of course, it was too much to expect men who had only a short while before been caught up in the horrors of war to be able to forget it and behave with respect towards the patients.
>
> (Nolan 1989: 59)

Nurses who felt undervalued and unsupported vented frustrations on clients without being detected, or challenged, by management.

Marginalised masculinities and health

The experiences of gay men with HIV and AIDS illustrate the complex ways in which gender constructions can affect health-related behaviours. Gay masculinities are marginalised masculinities; societal homophobia has led to gay men seeking status within their own communities. As Tewksbury (1995) notes, 'one of the most easily accessed, and for some most desirable, ways to pursue success has been to pursue an elusive goal of physical attractiveness and accumulated sexual conquests' (p. 228). The emphasis on sex and on physical attractiveness as an important part of gay identity can, therefore, be seen as a response to homophobic exclusion from other status-enhancing strategies. The inhibiting effects of HIV and AIDS on gay men's sexual activity can, therefore, lead to loss of status, self-esteem, and masculinity as well as physical and emotional intimacy. The reduction in sexual activity may derive from physical factors such as numbness, the side effects of medicines, a perceived decline in physical attractiveness and a loss of opportunities for sexual conquest, as well as from the changing meaning of sex through both the adoption of safe sex practices and changes in relationships.

Gay men with HIV and AIDS may reconstruct core elements of their identity through seeking new ways of establishing self-esteem as well as friendship and intimacy (Tewksbury 1995). The largely successful promotion of safe sex practices has been achieved through presenting the condom as consistent with a positively valued sexualised and hypermasculine gay identity (Wilton 1997). A deepening realisation of the possible fatal consequences of sexual activity has led to many HIV-positive gay men rethinking and restructuring their sexual lives, including adopting celibacy as a preventive measure, out of concern for others. Tewksbury (1995) notes the irony that living with HIV completely changes the meaning of sexual activity for a group of men defined by their sexual behaviour. HIV-positive gay men come to have very different lives from those without the disease.

Some of the successful methods of coping with HIV and AIDS adopted by the gay community are similar to the methods advocated by feminists for promoting women's health. Sharing experiences and mutual support networks as well as romantic relationships between men who are HIV-positive derives from the view that 'the complex emotional and social dynamics can only be fully appreciated by someone who has HIV disease' (Tewksbury 1995: 224). Such a view presents enormous challenges to any health professional since it suggests it is the clients and not the professionals, who best understand health and illness. What clients understand is not necessarily the physiological disease processes but their own lived experience of illness.

Nevertheless, some key features of gender-sensitive care are emerging. Sharing experience, developing non-hierarchical relationships and ensuring that patients and clients are well informed can help individuals to make sense of the effects of ill health on their lives and their gender roles. Factors that promote gender-sensitive care may include empathy and an orientation to others' needs, factors associated with femininity. Factors that inhibit supportive health care include the passivity and frustrations of oppressed groups. Nursing and nurses may well have suffered from the passivity of disempowered femininity and the bullying of frustrated and aggressive masculinity, features of a gendered culture that has devalued care. If nurses have suffered through a gendered culture, patients have suffered too. The interplay between gender, health and care is explored more fully in the following chapters through looking at gender, health and identity; gender, the body and sexuality; and gender, health and power.

10 Gender, identity and health

Introduction

This chapter looks at ways in which cultural constructions of masculinity and femininity can affect individual identity to the extent of damaging individual health and wellbeing. As noted in Chapter 6, masculinity has been associated with an autonomous, agentic self, and dependency has been seen as a feature of feminine roles. Adolescence is a period during which developing individual identities are particularly vulnerable to the possible negative consequences of dominant masculinities and femininities. Young men have high rates of accidents and self-destructive behaviour; young women have high rates of eating disorder. But gender roles and gendered identities can affect health throughout life. The salience of particular social roles (mother, financial provider) at different stages in individuals' lives may bring particular stresses for both men and women. The complex expectations associated with motherhood, for example, can lead to psychological difficulties including postnatal depression.

For some individuals, the effects of chronic illness can threaten their gender identity, that is, their self-perception of being male or female. For others, the experience of health care can threaten their personal identity. In a study of dissatisfaction with health care, Coyle (1999) found that 40 out of 41 respondents constructed accounts of their experience of care showing that they felt their identity had been undermined. 'Threats to personal identity included perceptions of being *dehumanised, objectified, stereotyped, disempowered* and *devalued*' (Coyle 1999: 107).

Concepts of identity

In sociology, identity has been seen as something to be shaped and developed through interaction, through culture and through discourse. As Weeks (1991) argues,

> identity is not inborn, pregiven, or 'natural'. It is striven for, contested, negotiated, and achieved, often in struggles of the subordinated against the dominant. Moreover, it is not achieved just by an individual act of will, or discovered hidden in the recesses of the soul. It is put together in circumstances bequeathed by history, in collective experiences as much as by individual destiny.
>
> (p. 94)

Identities are about what we want to be and could be. Nonetheless, they remain historically determined by the categories through which we view the world. Wilton (1996) has argued that the polarity of gender allows heterosexuality as a social system (Wittig 1992) to oppress women. The polarity of gender and the dominance of the male gender within heterosexuality as a social system may place any individuals, genetically male or female, who seek a 'female' gender identity in danger of experiencing the health costs of reduced self-efficacy and self-confidence.

Gender identity, however, may not conform to genetic identity; that is, some individuals may 'feel' male even though they have female genetic characteristics. Sexual orientation and gender identity can be linked in different ways, as can gender identity and social/gender roles. Cultural expectations of the links between genders and social roles are undergoing considerable change, which may eventually facilitate a greater acknowledgement of genetic variation as well as variations in gender identity and sexual preferences. However, as Beemer (1996) points out, 'society has a strong investment in seeing gender within rigid categories' (p. 13). Maintaining a binary view of sex, sexual orientation, gender, gender identity and gender roles supports a variety of ideological projects identified in Chapter 2, including heterosexuality, patriarchy and capitalism. Societal responses to individuals who have difficulty aligning their genetic identity, gender identity and gender role, and do not conform to a culturally expected sexual orientation, can hinder their development of a positive sense of identity and lead to difficulties that damage their health. It is, however, more complicated than that: individuals who rigidly align their genetic, gender, sexual and sex-role identities may also damage their health if the expected behaviour associated with a prescribed role (such as 'breadwinner' or 'mother') leads to health costs.

Adolescence, femininity and eating disorders

Eating disorders can illustrate the difficulties of identity development in a gendered culture. Anorexia nervosa has been recognised since the 1870s, although a key 1973 text noted its rarity (Bruch 1973). Characteristics of Western culture, including changes in women's role and a preoccupation with appearance and weight, appear to be associated with a rise in prevalence, particularly among young females (Gordon 1990). Kenny (1991) suggested a one per cent prevalence among middle-class adolescent girls. Although the range of explanations offered for anorexia nervosa include the view that a disorder of hypothalamic function may play a role in its development (Russell 1977), culture, alongside family interaction patterns, is usually seen as playing a significant role.

Minuchin's analysis of family interaction linked to anorexic symptoms described overprotectiveness, rigidity, an emphasis on conformity and a lack of conflict resolution as processes of enmeshment that inhibited the development of an autonomous identity (Minuchin et al. 1979). Bruch (1973, 1978) considered the relationship between mothers and daughters to be crucial and noted that the mothers of girls with anorexia nervosa had often relinquished their own career aspirations for family responsibilities. They had high expectations and aspirations for their daughters, leading to an emphasis on high academic achievement. The consequences for their daughters included difficulties distinguishing their own needs from those of their parents, an excessive concern about the feelings of others and a constant struggle for an independent identity. Lawrence (1987) noted, additionally, that a stress on the importance of education for women could set up conflicts for young women through apparently limiting the importance of motherhood. For young girls unwilling to face the conflicts, restricting weight gain inhibits normal development; a young girl remains a child.

Bruch argued that mothers' transference of their own ambitions onto their daughters while failing to encourage their daughters' own senses of identity resulted in the daughter's inability to differentiate between her own needs and those of others. This led to an inability to discriminate between hunger and feeling sated. An analysis of family dynamics led to family therapy as a form of treatment. However, Bruch's ideas also led to feminist approaches to understanding eating disorders.

Feminist approaches have stressed the importance of women's role in preparing food in Western cultures and the importance of women's roles as nurturer and as object of desire. Busfield (1996) notes that 'it is the convergence of women's focus on nurture and body image' (p. 180) that may lead to an emphasis on slimness as an expression of concern to give to others and meet standards of attractiveness for herself. Orbach (1993) argues that all eating disorders (anorexia, bulimia and obesity) should be understood in the context of patriarchal power, which has rendered women's own needs illegitimate. A control over food, including self-denial and rejection, is an 'attempt at empowering' (Orbach 1993: 83), an attempt to establish autonomy and a sense of self. Orbach's analysis, however, has been criticised for generalising too readily about the nature of women, ignoring the complexity of interpersonal relations and using a restricted analysis of the complexity of cultural influences.

Bordo (1990) identifies consumer capitalism as an additional source of cultural conflict. In consumer capitalism, we both produce and consume. Slenderness is both an ideal of female attractiveness, rendering women an object of male desire, and a symbol, for women, of liberation from the demands of domestic reproductive identities. Bordo suggests that control over body size can be seen as a means of embodying qualities associated with masculinity – detachment, self-containment, self-mastery and control. In achieving an extreme of femininity, women demonstrate an inner control over their lives (and their identity).

All explanations note that conflict and confusion surrounding societal, cultural and familial expectations over gender roles and gender identities are likely to be implicated in the development of eating disorders.

Eating disorders and nursing care

The treatment approach and nursing care for patients with anorexia nervosa have reflected different theoretical assumptions about the causative factors. Family therapy was the preferred treatment for many years; individual disordered patterns of control over eating habits were seen as deriving from feelings of being controlled by other family members. Characteristics of a family therapy approach include encouraging family members to explore possible reasons for behaviour and expressed feelings. The individual with an eating disorder is encouraged to explore his or her feelings towards family members and towards him- or herself. Behaviour and feelings can be reconsidered and reinterpreted with a view to developing different patterns of communication and relationships.

Although nurses may not have been extensively involved in family therapy or psychotherapy, nursing care, whatever the treatment regime, seeks to establish a relationship of trust, consistency, empathy and acceptance. Such a relationship challenges the nurse to explore his or her own thoughts and feelings about 'normal' and acceptable behaviour and relationships, and about mechanisms for coping with conflict. Anorexia nervosa can be accompanied by unproductive coping mechanisms such as obsessive-compulsive behaviour, secretiveness, delusional body image, depression, anxiety and suicidal tendencies.

Feminisms' interest in eating disorders has led to a woman-centred approach. Cowan (1996) criticises traditional psychiatric approaches for women as being 'based on helping them to adapt to social circumstances and to view their identity in terms of success in predetermined, societally dictated roles as wife, mother and sexual companion' (pp. 20–1). Woman-centred therapeutic approaches have adopted self-help, reciprocal, participatory approaches that enhance women's awareness of the ways in which women's perspective may have been subsumed under a narrow world view in which 'male values dominate and are the norm' (Cowan 1996: 22). Women can be encouraged to recognise the processes of oppression whereby the subordinate group internalise the norms and values of the oppressors so that they devalue themselves, unable to face the resulting, but suppressed, conflicts (Roberts 1983, Valentine 1992). A woman-centred therapeutic strategy in mental health aims at strengthening self-esteem, problem solving ability, autonomy and assertiveness.

Self-esteem in adolescence can be particularly negatively affected by the responses of caregivers, by social comparisons concerning physical appearance and by educational attainment. There is growing concern about changing gender roles at the end of the twentieth century having negative consequences for adolescent boys, but negative self-image has hitherto been more commonly associated with females than with males, as illustrated particularly through the prevalence of eating disorders among young women. Advice about goals of nursing care warrant careful scrutiny for assumptions that may lead to unintentionally limited support for a client whose eating disorder may stem from identity struggles associated with cultural assumptions about sexual orientation or about gender roles. Murray and Heulskoetter (1983), for example, identify nursing goals including 'social relationships with peers which demonstrate normal behaviour development'. The assumptions that lie behind a nurse's definition of normal behaviour development may not, however, necessarily be therapeutically helpful to an individual who does not, for example, seek 'normal' heterosexual relationships.

White (1991) advocates the demedicalisation of disordered eating through identifying a continuum of eating behaviours, thus broadening our perception of normality. 'Demedicalisation of those with disordered eating will occur if more information related to eating, diet, and weight management in a population of women who view themselves as healthy is provided' (White 1991: 77). She also criticises too ready an acceptance of the view that eating disorders are associated with low self-esteem. She reports a study in which obese women had high self-esteem despite a negative body image (White and Schroeder 1986). Women's increased involvement in exercise also contributes to the difficulty that some women have in maintaining body weight, introducing more variables into the links between culture, food, gender and eating disorders (Long and Hollin 1995).

Sloan (1999) advocates a cognitive-behavioural approach to the treatment of anorexia nervosa. The success of such an approach depends on developing a collaborative relationship between therapist and client, fostered through the therapist's warmth, honesty, empathy, courteousness and positive approach. On the basis of collaborative trust and through Socratic questioning, a nurse can enable the client to identify dysfunctional thoughts, which can be successfully challenged through cognitive restructuring techniques. Alternative ways of thinking bring the client the ability to change behaviour and develop a more optimistic and effective approach towards maintaining body weight. McGown and Whitbread (1996), in a review of studies of the effectiveness of treatment for bulimia nervosa, found that cognitive-behavioural therapy significantly reduced bingeing and purging episodes. 'What distinguishes the cognitive-behavioural approach from other techniques is its holistic view of the person, combining behavioural techniques, and addressing the cognitive elements, emotions, and interpersonal relations in a social environment' (McGown and Whitbread 1996: 35).

Gender dysphoria

Some individuals face extreme difficulties aligning their sense of who they are to their culturally prescribed gender identity. 'Gender identity disorder' is defined as being characterised by a persistent desire to be the opposite sex and by persistent and significant distress. Walters and Whitehead (1997) suggest that anxiety about developing male sexuality may be implicated in the development of anorexia among young men. The young boy whose case they discuss wanted to be a girl and thus faced a conflict between his wish to gain social acceptance through conforming to expected male behaviour and his revulsion at his developing male sexuality.

For some individuals, their genetic identity comes to be seen as incompatible with their preferred gender identity, leading to their identification as transsexual and to treatment for sexual realignment to conform to their chosen gender identity. Beemer (1996) notes the importance of ensuring that holistic care for patients undergoing gender transition is sensitive to the impediments they face. These impediments relate to the difficulties of their medical and surgical treatment, including their temporary physical and emotional state during a changing course of hormonal and surgical treatment, to the prevailing social milieu and to clinicians' assumptions about sexuality. Professionals involved in the care of transsexuals can be inappropriately and morbidly curious, partly in a misguided attempt to educate themselves. Beemer reminds nurses of the importance of acknowledging the self-chosen identity of the patient, empathising with the difficulties precipitated by hormonal change, monitoring progress, making appropriate referrals to other professionals for support and advice, and providing consistent, non-judgmental care and support. The provision of practical information, the avoidance of power struggles and ensuring that the patient takes the lead in decision making helps to ensure sensitive care.

Masculinity and identity

Chapter 3 has already explored links between mortality and masculinity. Young men have the highest rate of accidents, particularly motor vehicle accidents. This may reflect feelings of being in control and self-confidence, more negative masculine characteristics such as aggression, competitiveness and fear of subordination to another (particularly women), and gender neutral characteristics such as inexperience. The excitement of speed, of risk taking, and the feeling of physical indestructibility are all valued in male cultures. It is easy to see how traumatic damage to young men through accidents, alcohol and substance abuse may be linked to expectations of male behaviour, and to see young men as being particularly vulnerable to the hazards of conformity to masculine norms while developing their own sense of identity. The cultural influence of Freud's theories of masculine identity has played a role in reasserting a male concern for power and control. A small boy resolves his Oedipus complex – his love of his mother and his fear of his murderous feelings towards his powerful rival, his father – through relinquishing his primary identification with his mother in favour of identification with his father and all that his father represents: the male culture (Freud 1977, 1984).

Masculinity and sports injury

Sport is important in male culture. White *et al.* (1995) suggest that sport 'is intimately connected to gendering processes and argue that male involvement in physically hazardous sports is taken for granted, considered natural, and even appealing' (p. 158). Disregard for health in violent sports reinforces images of male omnipotence portrayed, for example, through films starring Arnold Schwarzenegger or Sylvester Stallone. White *et al.* (1995) link the valuing of a forceful masculinity through sport and leisure to the 'declining significance of male physicality in the sphere of work' (p. 159). Whereas a tolerance of male violence in many areas of life is decreasing, confrontational sport retains popularity in the media and remains strongly associated with masculinity.

The negative consequences for male athletes in terms of risk of injury, the occurrence of injury, rehabilitation, recovery and the possible long-term effects can be seen as the consequences of gendered forces resulting in physical hazards 'which are nevertheless naturalised, idealised and legitimised' (White *et al.* 1995: 161). Messner (1990) has noted the way in which socialisation into seeing bodies as 'machines and weapons with which to annihilate an objec-tified opponent, ultimately comes back upon the athlete as an alien force' (p. 211). When the machine-like body is damaged and in pain, it may be experienced as alien. White *et al.*'s study of 16 athletes identified that all had experienced considerable pain and multiple injuries. In addition, all associated masculinity, identity and sport; sport helped to establish 'a robust and competent physical sense of self' (White *et al.* 1995: 166). Sport also reproduced 'dominance bonding' (Farr 1988), a system of peer group-based male privilege developed through the locker room culture and through the shared responsibility for team success. A motivation to ignore pain when injured develops in response to group processes through which an injured player is defined as deviant. Returning to sport after an injury and enduring the pain of an injury is seen as restoring mental and physical strength and reconstructing masculinity. 'The battle-worn athlete is subjectively hypermasculine when objectively he may be physically disabled' (White *et al.* 1995: 177). In such circumstances, hearing medical caution and advice can be difficult: 'several subjects spoke of being bewildered by the ominous prognoses of doctors cautioning them against repeated risk taking' (p. 175). Changing sportsmen's behaviour may involve reconstructing identity through changing attitudes to risk.

Hearn (1998) argues that understanding men's identity in the social context involves recognising that men's identity usually includes an acceptance of men's power relationship over women. 'The psychological and social identity called "man" says and shows power relations' (p. 4). Men's violence towards themselves, which is one way of seeing men's damage to their own health, may be a form of exerting power in order to avoid a feeling of inferiority or loss of control.

Masculinity and suicidal acts

There is considerable concern that young men in Britain are increasingly troubled by feelings of inferiority and that their response is a masculine one: to seek power and control through behaviour that damages their own and others' health. Whereas male mortality rates in England and Wales for accidents, poisoning and violence have decreased in all social classes from 1970, mortality from suicide and undetermined injury has increased in all social classes except social class I. Death rates for unskilled workers (social class V) have increased from 32 per 100,000 in 1970–72 to 47 per 100,000 in 1991–93 (Drever and Bunting 1997, Acheson 1998). Suicide rates are highest of all among the unemployed. The increase in suicidal behaviour among men, in particular young men, is now attracting research and policy interest. The Green Paper *Our Healthier Nation* (DoH 1998a) suggests that a possible target for the reduction of suicide rate could be to reduce the death rate from suicide and undetermined injury by one sixth by 2010 from a baseline of 1996. Our understanding of male suicide, attempted suicide and self-harm, however, remains limited.

Hitherto, in Britain and the United States, although men engaged in fewer suicidal acts than women, men's suicide attempts were more likely to be successful. Canetto (1992–93, 1995) argues that, in the United States, surviving a suicidal act is 'unmasculine', and men are most critical of other men who fail to take their own life, seeing such behaviour as violating male norms of 'strength, decisiveness, success and inexpressiveness' (White and Stillion 1988). Men are seen as suicidal because of health- or work-related problems rather than relationship failure. Hence, as Canetto (1995) notes, research has concentrated on the relationship between suicidal behaviour and work roles, to the neglect of interpersonal factors.

Thus, gendered assumptions may distort patterns of enquiry and limit the information we have. Furthermore, the information collected on suicidal acts is itself subject to variations in reporting and recording practices. Male suicidal behaviour may have been underreported in the past; more public concern may lead to greater public acceptability and changes in patterns of reporting and diagnosing self-destructive acts.

Depression is widely reported as a risk factor for suicide, and an increase in the prevalence of depression among men might help to explain the rise in male suicide rate. Shajahan and Cavanagh (1998) found a rise in the rate of admission for depression to Scottish hospitals for men from 1980 to 1995 and a decrease in the rate of admission for depression among women, although women continued to have a higher rate than men. The authors suggest that this may be because of changes in gender roles, a decrease in the number of men in full-time work and a rise in the number of women in part-time and full-time work. 'For men the resultant loss of status as sole financial provider for the family, the perceived loss in social status, and the consequent social isolation could all be considered risk factors for depression' (p. 1497). Nevertheless, Shajahan and Cavanagh also note that the rise in admission rate may reflect an increase in the number of men being referred by their general practitioner, a change in admission criteria, an increased recognition of depression and a change in men's help seeking behaviour. An increase in attempted suicide or deliberate self-harm may, similarly, not necessarily reflect a 'real' change in levels of distress among men but could reflect changes in ways of signalling that distress. The rise in successful suicide, however, suggests that the rise in distress is real and that men's response can still be decisive and effective.

Male suicide can also be prompted by a rigid inability to tolerate the uncertainty that derives from changing gender roles and changes in masculine roles of dominance and independence. Canetto (1995), in a review of the literature on male suicidal acts, notes that, for some men, 'an external loss such as retirement or a minor physical disability... may be uniquely stressful because it threatens their sense of masculinity' (p. 302). This has been found to be particularly the case among older men who kill themselves (Clark 1993). For other men, external losses may be less significant than interpersonal ones. Canetto concludes that 'a shift in their gender identity and assumptions could be a key to their survival. A focus on gender can thus broaden possibilities for the prevention of male suicidal behaviour' (p. 302).

Motherhood and postnatal depression

Not only can difficulties developing a 'normal' male identity bring health risks, but so too can achieving the exemplar of female-gendered status – motherhood. Motherhood is presented as a 'natural' state for women, and reactions to motherhood are often judged by lay assumptions about 'maternal instincts', reinforced by theory and research in psychology that has explored the process of mother–infant bonding. The work of Klaus and Kennell (1976), which suggested that 'bonding' was particularly easy between 6 and 12 hours after birth and could be facilitated by skin-to-skin contact between mother and baby, led to changes in hospital access policies for mothers and babies (Littlewood and McHugh 1997). Subsequent research concerning attachment theory has led to a recognition of the importance of the quality of relationships between caregivers and infants; however, myths about natural motherhood have led to generalised assumptions about the ease with which 'normal' women adjust to motherhood. Good women, good mothers and motherhood epitomise naturalised femininity. As Littlewood and McHugh (1997) point out, Christian ideology supported a link between virtue and motherhood through the importance of the Virgin Mary. In Britain, in times when Christian ideology dominated cultural life, any negative reaction to motherhood had to be managed in private; there was little public discourse about what is now regarded as depression following birth of a child. 'It was only when the physical problems associated with childbirth were finally almost completely overcome by antibiotics and blood transfusions that postnatal depression began to be recognised as a problem in its own right' (Littlewood and McHugh 1997: 16).

Bewley (1999) distinguishes between baby blues, puerperal psychosis and postnatal depression. Holden (1990) estimates that between 50 and 70 per cent of new mothers experience the baby blues. Puerperal psychosis is a rare, serious psychiatric disorder developing in the first week after childbirth. Postnatal depression, which about 10 per cent of mothers, although estimates vary, may experience over a variable period, manifests itself up to six months postpartum. Women who are depressed during the early stages of motherhood may experience a range of symptoms including anxiety, panic attacks, tension and irritability, depression, exhaustion, lack of concentration, loss of libido, feelings of rejection, sleep and appetite disturbance, exhaustion and obsessional or negative thoughts about the baby (Bewley 1999). Women may also experience considerable difficulty acknowledging and seeking help for their distress because of the social construction of motherhood as a positive and desirable identity.

The causes of postnatal depression are debated. Dalton (1985) has argued that some women are particularly sensitive to hormonal changes, particularly the rise in progesterone level, post-childbirth. Dalton advocated progesterone prophylactic treatment for women identified as being 'at risk', but research has not confirmed the efficacy of progesterone (Vandermeer *et al.* 1984). Gregoire *et al.* (1996), in a small study of postnatally depressed women, found that oestrogen significantly improved mood. Birth trauma, 'a fundamental negative birth experience that may be either physical or psychological in origin' (Littlewood and McHugh 1997: 38), has been identified as a possible cause. Trauma often results from a combination of physical and psychological factors; the physical intervention, ranging from episiotomy to emergency caesarean section, may be perceived as unnecessary, inappropriate or a violation of the woman's body (Kitzinger 1992, Kendall-Thackett and Kaufman-Kanter 1993).

Feminist writers see the trauma that women may experience during the process of giving birth as the trauma of powerlessness. During childbirth, women may feel a loss of control and a sense of betrayal or abuse by the professionals trusted to care for them during the delivery. If the delivery is 'abnormal', women may feel stigmatised (Kendall-Thacket and Kaufman-Kanter 1993). Ussher (1991) suggests that 'postnatal depression' is a label that serves the interests of a patriarchal society; it serves to identify women as being deviant, unnatural mothers. As such, it is not a label that health professionals should readily adopt.

It is the losses that women may experience on becoming a mother that can change women's lives significantly in ways that may lead to feelings of isolation and depression. Despite the idealisation of motherhood it can, for mothers in the late twentieth century, be an isolating experience during which women may suffer temporary or permanent loss of employment, loss of status, loss of personal and financial independence, loss of privacy and loss of social support and social networks (Oakley 1979). Such losses may result in the loss of a sense of personal identity, accompanied by the confusing experience of the reality of motherhood. Charles and Walters (1998) quote a mother's description of her feelings during postnatal depression:

> I can't cope... I haven't been able to cope as I used to like... and I don't want to be the person I've turned into, you know what I mean, nagging and crying all the time... I just feel like running away... because I don't want to be this mother and the wife I am at the moment. (05M – 24 years)
>
> (p. 342)

For many women whose financial and social circumstances are such that caring for their children is exceedingly difficult, a sense of hopelessness may lead to the loss of a sense of value and reward. Brown and Harris' (1978) important study on women and depression noted 'that what is important about such loss for the genesis of depression is that it leads to an inability to hold good thoughts about ourselves, our lives and those close to us' (p. 233). From an analytical standpoint that views motherhood in the context of a patriarchal society, maternal depression is widespread, associated with the cultural oppression of mothers and women. Nicolson (1986) argues that depression can become a period of reflection during which women re-evaluate their roles, aspirations and relationships. The arrival of a baby may lead to a recognition of the oppressive nature of women's relationships or circumstances, including difficulties for women in the employment market. Symonds and Hunt (1996) suggest that, on motherhood, some women simply wish to mourn the loss of a previous lifestyle and previous identity, but with no culturally sanctioned 'lying in' period, 'there is no time to mourn the life that has past; only the work of the new' (p. 116). The work of the new may still involve the responsibility for the care of child and household within a gendered culture that continues to segregate men's and women's work. Charles and

Walters (1998) found that in a South Wales working-class community characterised by

> changing gender relations, male unemployment... and a lack of support to enable younger women to combine parenting with employment... the stress younger women reported arose from the gender and class relations within which they were located, which meant that they had the responsibility of managing a family on low and precarious incomes.

> (p. 347)

Gordon (1998) illustrates the importance of the cultural context of motherhood in a study of influences on mothers' breastfeeding decisions. Women's choice of feeding approach depends on the configuration of the roles that women are able to play in any society. Gordon's study of infant feeding methods in County Antrim in 1993, for example, revealed the extent to which women's attitudes to breastfeeding were consonant with those of their partners. Partners in favour of artificial feeding saw breastfeeding mothers as being assertive, 'forward' and 'showie'. 'Partners with children being breastfed saw breastfeeding mothers as confident, caring and self-assertive' (Gordon 1998: 164). Gordon notes that the responsibility for empowering a mother to make a choice about infant feeding involves much more than giving information; it also involves understanding the political, economic and cultural forces that shape women's lives, and working together to remove some of the barriers to women's ability to choose their own approaches to mothering.

Professional strategies to support mothers

Women probably have more contact with health professionals during pregnancy and the early postnatal period than at any other time during their lives. Midwives, general practitioners and health visitors are all involved in the care of mothers and infants, but if a woman is perceived as distressed or depressed, psychiatric nurses, psychiatrists and other professionals may become involved. A feminist social science analysis may suggest that a preferable response to postnatal depression would be to normalise it; research suggests that women do not wish to be identified as not coping with motherhood. McIntosh (1993) found low levels of help seeking behaviour among depressed women. Whitton *et al.* (1996), in a survey of 78 mothers with postnatal depression, found that only 12 per cent had spoken to a health professional. Women who may have had negative feelings about their experience of birth are unlikely to seek the support of health professionals. However, the government Green Paper *Supporting Families* (DoH 1998b) suggests that midwives and health visitors could play a role in improving family relationships.

Professional concern about identifying unmet need has to be tempered by an awareness that increased professional intervention into personal lives can be part of a creeping medicalisation that reduces parents' ability to help themselves and their families. Successful intervention strategies, however, adopt collaborative, supportive and non-interference principles. Holden (1990) noted that health visitors trained in non-directive counselling techniques and using the Edinburgh Postnatal Depression Scale (EPDS) could effectively improve the mood of depressed mothers. Holden (1994) argues that use of the EPDS, a short 10-item questionnaire, gives women and professionals the opportunity to reflect on emotional responses and alert women to the nature of support available from health professionals. Littlewood and McHugh (1997) see the EPDS as an effective and efficient screening tool that can be used to identify a need for service provision and to encourage interdisciplinary collaboration. A multidisciplinary strategy in Oxford, using the EPDS as a validated assessment strategy, led to a collaborative, client-centred approach in which participants worked flexibly across professional boundaries.

Oates (1988) reports on a scheme in Nottingham in which community psychiatric nurses acted as key workers for women with severe postnatal depression, flexibly deploying the resources of the community, family and other members of the psychiatric team. Oates saw this integrated community scheme as being an alternative to day hospital facilities.

Current policy initiatives and suggestions to target support for mothers as a means of improving community health may lead to a greater use of voluntary services in conjunction with health professionals, and greater attention being paid to prevention strategies. The Association for Post Natal Illness and Meet-a-Mum Association both provide information as well as group and one-to-one support for depressed women and their families. They encourage women to see postnatal depression as an illness and to seek help, and urge families to recognise that mothers need rest and practical support. Charles and Curtis (1994) discuss the concept of post-delivery debriefing as a means of giving women the opportunity to discuss their experience of labour with a view to preventing the development of emotional difficulties. Skilled and empathetic professionals continue to explore ways of supporting women as they grow accustomed to their identity as a mother (Littlewood and McHugh 1997). The ability to empathise, however, depends on an understanding of the conditions of women's lives.

Chronic illness and identity

The achievement-orientated values of modern Western cultures are best achieved by a healthy population (Bury 1997). Individuals, and society, emphasise a view of illness as temporary and episodic, under the control of professionals and patients, playing their parts in enacting and supporting the 'sick role' (Parsons 1951). The experience of chronic illness, however, 'fractures this social and cultural fabric, exposing the individual to threats of self-identity and a potentially damaging loss of control' (Bury 1997: 124).

Bury (1982, 1991) sees chronic illness as a 'biographical disruption'; changes to the body and experiences of the body change an individual's social situation and affect relationships. Bury (1997) suggests that it is the meaning of chronic illness in terms of its *consequences* and *significance* that affects individual biographies. Symptoms have practical and social consequences that have to be managed; these symptoms and their disabling effects will vary in significance for the individuals concerned, depending on societal response to the condition itself and on the challenges to the individual's identity. Bury (1997) suggests that 'biographical disruption can be mitigated in at least two ways: efforts may be made to construct a reasonable level of *explanation* for the illness and to establish its *legitimacy* in the person's life' (p. 125). Health and social care professionals, through providing treatment and care, play a key role in the process of explaining and legitimising a chronic condition within a person's biography. A range of sociological studies have illuminated this process from the client's perspective. Kelleher (1988) has written about diabetes, Robinson (1988) about multiple sclerosis, Williams (1993) about chronic respiratory disease, and Williams *et al.* (1996) about arthritis.

The process of adaptation and negotiation through which individuals face the challenges of chronic illness involves active responses that Bury (1991) has summarised as *coping*, *strategy* and *style*. *Coping* refers to problem-based and emotional-based coping. *Strategy* is a term used to acknowledge attempts to mobilise resources in support of self and illness management, whereas *style* is the 'performance' undertaken with other people in mind. Bury's analysis draws on the insights of interactionist and social constructionist approaches in sociology, which offer individuals some choice and control over their own identity construction and life meaning. Nevertheless, he notes the importance of socioeconomic status, particularly in relation to the strategies available to individuals in managing chronic conditions. 'The term "strategy" brings the 'rules and resources' of social hierarchies' (Bury 1997: 131) into focus. Individual energy and effort are important resources but so too are material factors such as income and housing, as well as social relationships providing practical and social support.

British research into the management of chronic illness and the effect of illness on identity has not paid much attention to gender differences and the effects of gender on coping, strategy and style. American literature shows interest in masculinity. Charmaz (1991, 1995) studied identity dilemmas for chronically ill men through in-depth interviews with 20 adult men, making a comparison with 80 interviews with chronically ill women. Charmaz (1995) notes that the biographical disruptions for men tend to be more sudden and more serious than for women. Women experience more progressive, degenerative disease such as arthritis and multiple sclerosis. Men have more and earlier heart attacks and strokes. Illness can create a domino effect of identity losses:

> chronic illness can alter or end men's participation in work, sports, leisure, and sexual activities. Hence illness can reduce a man's status in masculine hierarchies, shift his power relations with women, and raise his self-doubts about masculinity.
>
> (Charmaz 1995: 268)

Charmaz identifies four main experiences: 'awakening to death after a life threatening crisis'; 'accommodating to uncertainty'; 'defining illness and disability'; and 'preserving self to maintain a sense of coherence while experiencing loss and change'. Awakening to death can be a profound shock to men who perceive themselves as fit and healthy, and too young to die. Methods of coping include treating illness as a set of problems to solve and finding new meanings and legitimation in their social roles in the family, made possible through the ease with which men are able to rely on the supportive response of their families. Charmaz (1995) reports that

> they received an outpouring of care, comfort and love from their wives and families. These men often bragged about how supportive and helpful their wives had been. Even men who had troubled marriages felt their wives affirmed, valued and supported them.
>
> (p. 272)

Men's initial attempts to maintain control over uncertainty were characterised by continuing to see themselves as risk takers and winners or seeing the onset of heart disease as something they would recover from, able to return to their former activities. With increasing recognition that their bodies have changed, reappraisal is possible.

Reappraisal, involving their own way of accommodating to uncertainty, gave some men a clearer awareness of their identity. A process of reassessment could involve differing definitions of their illness or disability, objectifying it as an enemy or as an ally, seeing it as an intrusive presence or as an opportunity. Viewing illness as an intrusive presence or as an opportunity integrated the bodily changes into self-conception, which seemed to be easier for older men. Middle-aged and younger men frequently invoked the 'competitive discourse of victories and losses when talking about their illness' (p. 276).

Charmaz found that some of the younger and middle-aged men took years to recognise the identity dilemmas that illness and disability posed them. They made use of resources available through work, physique and family relationships to maintain a sense of control. Being able to control the conditions and logistics of work (office location and hours worked) made it easier for some middle-class men to preserve their sense of identity; others went to considerable lengths to control their public presentation of self, through, for example, ceasing to go to the canteen when unable to manage a wheelchair and a tray. Some allowed illness and disability to 'engulf' them at home, becoming tyrannical and self-pitying patients but thereby maintaining some control in the domestic sphere. Charmaz concludes that since visible disability reduces men's position in the hierarchy of men, men have a greater stake in preserving their past identities than do women. Older, working-class men, however, were more resigned and more able to build their lives around illness.

Charles and Walters' (1998) accounts of South Wales women's response to arthritis support the view that women accommodate chronic illness, together with the accompanying hardships, into their lives more readily than men. The older women in their study regarded arthritis as natural, normal and familiar. Women rarely sought medical help despite the restrictions that arthritis placed on their activities. Arthritis was seen as an inevitable part of growing older and could be managed by adapting their domestic routines.

Anderson *et al.* (1997) have reported on the effect of arthritis on women's employment, noting that 'working double shifts in physically demanding jobs and managing housework typifies the lives of many women' (p. 63). They researched the experiences of Chinese women living in Canada. The effect of illness on family wellbeing caused the women distress, and their circumstances made it difficult for them to put their own health first. Despite the effect of material circumstances on their response to illness and vice versa, the centrality of women's caring roles may mean that chronic illness, especially of a progressive, degenerative nature, may not disrupt women's biographies as significantly as men's. Anderson *et al.* (1997), recognising health professionals' privileged position in hearing the stories of women's lives, argue that professionals should understand 'the histories that have shaped the lives of different groups' and accept the challenge of working towards justice for all people (p. 76).

Nurses are increasingly accepting the challenge of understanding patients' lived experience of illness. This is usually presented as enhancing the uniqueness of the individual caring relationship rather than as contributing to working for justice. Clare Hastings' account of caring for a women with arthritis whom she met briefly in a rheumatology screening clinic is used by Benner and Wrubel (1989) to illustrate the primacy of caring. The woman's disease was advanced. Clare Hastings' familiarity with the symptoms enabled her to demonstrate her understanding: 'It looks like you haven't been able to use this hand for a long time.' She could ask questions about practical ways of coping with the disease: 'Does anyone help you get dressed in the morning?' It was clear that the woman had received and asked for little help. The nurse noted 'she had gone through many years of what I considered almost useless suffering'. The empathy implicit in the questioning and in the examination prompted tears; 'no one has ever talked to me as if this were a thing that mattered, a personal event'. Understanding the personal nature of the lived experience of illness reduced the 'isolation and suffering created by the disease' (Benner and Wrubel 1989: 11). Although nursing literature rarely discusses the lived experience of illness as a gendered experience, it does illuminate the importance of nurses listening and hearing (sometimes through touch) and seeking justice through the intimacy of nursing care. I suggest that Clare Hastings was listening to a gendered experience through which a woman demonstrated both strength and passivity (characteristics of a 'good woman'), through chronic suffering.

11 Gender, power and sexuality

Introduction

The intimacy of nursing care involves nurses in confronting the complexity of social taboos concerning our bodies. Western, particularly British, cultural traditions tend to be 'non-touching', and many nurses, as Lawler (1991) identified, report 'feeling terror, embarrassment and timidity when they first had to confront other people's nakedness, and at having to undress people, particularly men' (p. 119). Lawler notes that 'the relationship of maleness and male power to genitalia and sexuality had a powerful effect' (p. 118). She argues that 'male sexuality and masculinity are genital and physical constructs to a greater extent than is the case for female sexuality and femininity' (p. 195). Nurses have to find ways of managing male sexuality as they accomplish their nursing care. This chapter explores the health care implications of the power dimension in gender relations.

Care of the body and sexuality

Nurses manage their care of the body through controlling any indication of affective responses, retaining a 'professional' manner, working with speed and a 'matter-of-fact' approach. Nurses are also tolerant and accepting of the fact that care of the body can be a sensual experience, but they control attempts by patients to define situations as being primarily sexual. Breaking taken-for-granted rules through overt sexual behaviour can be controlled through jokes, humour and trivialising, but Lawler suggests that nurses have been silent about what can be construed as sexual harassment. As one of her respondents commented,

I think a lot probably goes on that goes unreported because nurses are afraid that they might be thought to be encouraging it or something... Nurses do not appreciate being mauled... It shouldn't be what we are expected to put up with.

(p. 210)

Lawler (1991) reports that orthopaedic patients were identified as 'stereotypically sexual harassers of nurses' (p. 211). It is commonplace for young male orthopaedic patients to make sexually suggestive comments; 'orthopaedic wards can resemble other male dominated situations where sex-as-sport forms part of the local culture' (p. 211). Lawler notes that sexual harassment in nursing is a heterosexual matter; heterosexuality pervades social life so extensively that it is not excluded from patient care. Homosexuality, however, is not so culturally overt; Lawler found that sexual advances made between patients and nurses of the same sex were (reportedly) rare (p. 213).

Parkin (1989) has argued that 'sexuality is an ever-present issue for workers and residents within residential care organisations, yet is notably absent from staff meeting agendas, training programmes, organisational policies, rules and guidelines' (p. 110). In a study of residential care workers, managers and CQSW students, she found that the inevitable intimacy and closeness of the work led to the organisation of work, such as the rotation of duties, being affected by an implicit consideration of connotations of sexuality without any explicit discussion between management and staff. There was, however, considerable informal discussion among lower-level staff, and students welcomed the opportunity to discuss problems and ambiguities. Male students and staff reported considerable caution in their behaviour with young people of either sex. At the time of her research, Parkin (1989) found very little management guidance on personal relationships between staff and residents; the individual's 'professionalism' was relied upon and was blamed as deficient if problems emerged, as they did. Parkin refers to national scandals and local incidents, including the sacking of a worker in a hostel for mentally ill people for having an affair with a resident.

Parkin's case material included an example of a high turnover of female staff in a residential unit with a husband and wife team in a managerial role. The husband arranged the staff rota in order to be on duty with targeted female staff. Complaints to higher managers were referred to the husband and wife team, with no action being taken. The management response, when the couple left, was to change procedures to prohibit the employment of a married couple. Parkin saw this example as illustrating the pervasive power of male domination; males dominate not only in private (sexual) relationships, but also in the public world of work. Residential care institutions occupy an intermediate zone between private and public worlds since they have characteristics of each. This intermediacy allows different approaches to the organisation and scrutiny of work. Some aspects of work, such as the control of sexuality in the context of the intimacy of care, are subject to informal guidance, rules and conventions. There appeared to be little attempt to develop protocols or appropriate methods of surveillance at management level.

Parkin's research indicated that 'issues around sexuality continued to be grievances for staff and residents alike, with both powerless to have them heard officially' (p. 117). Parkin describes management failure to deal with grievances as 'non-decision making' (Bachrach and Baratz 1962), an illustration of Lukes' (1974) second face of power in which issues are kept off the agenda. As a result, a culture of oppressive sexuality can remain unchallenged. Wardhaugh and Wilding (1993) have identified the 'neutralisation of normal moral concerns' as being one of eight elements in systems of organisation that they see as able to contribute to 'the corruption of care'. Other elements are: the balance of power and powerlessness; particular pressures and particular types of work; management failure; enclosed, inward-looking organisations; an absence of clear lines and mechanisms of accountability; particular models of work and organisation; and the nature of certain client groups. It is easy to see how sexuality can be part of the corruption of care.

Sensitivity to clients' perceptions of bodily care by male and female nurses and to clients' feelings of disempowerment through nursing and medical care is, however, demonstrated in nursing and health care literature. Lodge *et al.* (1997) studied gynaecological patients' perceived embarrassment with physical and psychological care given by male and female nurses and the relationship between the intimacy of a nursing procedure and the level of embarrassment. An analysis of 91 questionnaires indicated that female patients with no prior experience of hospital admission or of being cared for by a male nurse expressed a preference for care from a female nurse. However, patients with a hospital admission in the past five years or with an experience of care from a male nurse did not demonstrate such a preference. Women not in relationships were significantly less embarrassed by care given by a male nurse, suggesting that 'actual care may not be the issue. The issue could be how men are viewed as carers in our society. The female patient may not wish to displace her partner as the only male allowed to... be close to her' (Lodge *et al.* 1997: 902). McKie (1996) found examples of women taking account of their (male) partners' constructions of health care procedures in a study of women's talk about the cervical smear test. Women reported male partners' perceptions of the test as having the potential for sexual thrills and a widespread view that a positive smear is linked to promiscuity. Such views could inhibit women's attendance for smear tests.

Rhodes (1994), in a study of continence advisors, notes sensitivity concerning male and female nurses' involvement in vaginal examinations and male catheterisation. There has been a strong tradition that female nurses should not perform male catheterisations, although it is unclear whether this is a matter of skill, to protect female nurses or to reduce male embarrassment. Some nurses were concerned that vaginal examination could be regarded as a form of abuse. Increased sensitivity to changing definitions of abuse may have led to a redefinition of some procedures as the responsibility of specialists, rather than generalist community nurses. Changing definitions and increased sensitivity to the appropriateness of physical examinations and bodily care by men and women from different professional specialisms may derive from an increased recognition of the importance of the client's rights and feelings. Tiefer (1997), for example, commenting on her work as a psychologist in a urology clinic, describes how she attempts to counteract the medicalised approach to male sexual function by ensuring that partners' views are also listened to. She notes:

> In the urology setting women's interests are assumed to be central to the evaluation, the prime reason why the man is coming for treatment. Yet, women are usually omitted from the evaluation... My work has explicitly invited women to contribute as equal partners.

> (p. 111)

Few (1997) argues that nurses need to enhance their understanding of power issues involved in sexual activity and sexual health. General cultural difficulties in finding a language to describe and discuss sexual practices in terms that are neither clinical nor derogatory leads to difficulties in providing explicit, understandable details of, for example, the risk of HIV transmission. This leads to a poor understanding of the risk of HIV transmission in different sexual practices among young people (Macintyre and West 1993). Few warns against a reliance on methods aimed at promoting condom use that do not take account of the realities of women's power to change situations. If women are in a situation in which they have no power, asking male partners to use condoms may make them more vulnerable. Few encourages nurses to recognise that

> inequality of women in heterosexual relationships must be acknowledged... Decision-making about sexual behaviour involves cultural and sex role norms that may inhibit women from exercising freedom of choice. The self-esteem of women should be a concern of all health care professionals working in the area of sexual health. High self-esteem is necessary for assuming responsibility for decisions about sex and sexual relationships.
>
> (1997: 623)

Taylor (1995) identifies the importance of practice nurses recognising how gender-power relations may restrict their own role expansion through their employers' (general practitioners') role in providing in-service training. Many practice nurses providing family planning advice, for example, may not have received appropriate education, 'Yet even the recognised course reinforces the patriarchal ideology by focusing on the woman's reproductive role' (Taylor 1995: 691). Promoting safe sex involves promoting positive images of women and men as equals in sexual relationships.

Segal (1997) argues that feminism (the 'feminist polemic' as she describes it) has done little to open up discussion about sexuality; heterosexuality has been identified as the 'cause and enactment of men's power over women' and linked to male violence (p. 79). As a result of a feminist emphasis on women's disempowerment, Segal argues that heterosexual women have remained silent about their own sexual agency. Within the context of a culture that has little to say about the details of sexual behaviour, particularly female sexual behaviour, nursing's own reticence is not surprising.

Sexual identity and the experience of illness

The experience of diseases that may be perceived as affecting body image and sexuality has been explored in both nursing and social science literature. Gordon (1995), himself a testicular cancer survivor, studied men's experience of testicular cancer. Testicular cancer is the most common cancer in men between the ages of 20 and 34 and the second most common between the ages of 35 and 39 (ONS 1998b), a period during which men are developing careers and commitments to partners and children. Cure rates are high but treatment can affect fertility, involves the surgical removal of a testicle and can thus affect body image and sexual function.

From his interviews with 20 survivors, Gordon identified three major stages of adjustment. The first stage included an intense fear of death, disfigurement and suffering. This was followed by a process of working through what the experience of disease meant for their lives. Since the chance of survival was high, many men were able to adapt positively. Despite a change in body image, they were able to resume sexual activity and were often well supported by their wives. Thus, what appeared to be a threat to masculine identity in fact became an opportunity to reaffirm masculinity. In the third stage of adjustment to the disease, men drew on two different strategies to arrive at a set of meanings. One was a traditional masculine strategy, defining the experience as 'a serious fight in which they displayed courage in the face of fear' (Gordon 1995: 255). They handled emotion 'like men'. Although many did report negative body images, negative feelings were not dwelt upon: 'They attempted to deny or hide their feelings' (p. 257). Joking about the loss of a testicle, returning to previous activities, including physical activities, as quickly as possible and keeping feelings to themselves were common approaches. Gordon notes that this often left wives to 'do whatever emotional work needs to be done'. Men's inexpressiveness forced wives to concentrate on emotional issues (both their own and the family's).

An alternative or co-existing strategy was non-traditional, through which the experience of the disease enabled men to redefine their priorities, which led to the placing of an increased importance on personal relationships as well as to a greater awareness of personal suffering. However, none of the men questioned the idea of masculinity. Testicular cancer, despite affecting body image and appearing to threaten sexual function, is thus often experienced in a way in which masculine identity is reaffirmed. Jones and Webb (1994), in an interview study of 18 men treated for testicular cancer, found that concern for their survival took precedence over concerns about fertility or sexuality. The high rate of cure, therefore, encourages a positive view about beating the disease. However, one 20-year-old single man expressed deep concern about any possible recurrence of the cancer, leading to the loss of a second testicle. The possibility of not being able to have children was a major worry. Jones and Webb (1994) found that 'lack of information, misinformation and misunderstandings' were common themes in the men's interviews. Nurses' role in their care seemed relatively insignificant. Jones and Webb (1994) suggest that, given the difficulties that health care staff often experience in discussing sexuality with clients, the effective care of men with testicular cancer may be more successfully developed through a clinical nurse specialist role.

Specialist breast care nurses play a major role in the care of women with breast cancer. The importance of involving women in making choices about their own treatment has encouraged the development of the role of specialist breast care nurse to support women, particularly through supporting their information needs (Miers 1999b). Although changes in body image affect the experience of the disease, it is the chance of survival that is often the most important issues for those with cancer (Luker *et al.* 1993, 1996).

Colyer (1996) began her small study of women's experience of breast cancer assuming that the focus of women's concerns would be body image and sexuality, but she found that the locus of women's pain seemed 'to be more fundamentally related to existence itself'. Assumptions about 'being in the world' are threatened by the uncertainty of the disease. The changes in body image are associated with a disease that threatens life. Hence the societal stigma of the altered body image *and* of the unpredictability of life-threatening cancer combine to disrupt a woman's sense of identity. A patriarchal framing of images of womanhood, with its emphasis on particular images of sexual attractiveness, creates difficulties for women attempting to adjust to changing perceptions of both their vulnerability and their body image. The experience of illness, however, may lead to an increased recognition of possibilities of self-identities that are not constrained by hegemonic femininities (Colyer 1996).

Disempowerment through health care

Coyle (1999) suggests that the experience of health care as well as the experience of disease can be disempowering. For some patients, the resulting feelings of disempowerment could be the substance of a complaint. Coyle (1999) found that being treated as an object, stereotyped as being of low intelligence, infantile, incompetent or 'unbalanced', and having their condition misdiagnosed or ignored, often through being treated on the basis of age, were the main reasons for complaint, particularly for women. Coyle's respondents identified three types of disempowerment; through the way in which power was exerted over them, through the way in which power was taken from them, and through 'being unable to resist the definitions and labels of the dominant, in this case the medical and patriarchal discourses' (p. 115). For men, the loss of power to perform normal social roles was the main reason for feelings of disempowerment; women reported all three types of disempowerment. Feminist research has identified ways in which doctors can use and perpetuate negative stereotypes of women (Roberts 1985, Foster 1989, Miles 1991). Coyle (1999) found that, for the women in her study, 'a common consequence... was that they felt doctors had failed to listen, take their anxieties seriously or investigate the illness' (p. 112).

Lumby (1997) reports on her doctoral and post-doctoral work with a group of women experiencing end stage liver disease. A central theme for the women was that of control. Women experienced feelings of 'being in control', 'being out of control' and 'being controlled by others' throughout their health care, from diagnosis, through surgery to discharge. Lumby's study revealed many examples of women demonstrating their own control through prioritising families over illness. One woman who continued to work as a nurse felt so ill when preparing a birthday meal for her son in the evening that she went to bed, later to be found by her husband comatosed from liver failure. She had a transplant operation the following day. Other women reorganised their family's roles and activities to ensure that family members were relatively unaffected by their transplant surgery. 'One woman spoke of setting goals for herself in order to have a sense of control, while others planned their funeral services or celebrations in case they did not survive the transplantation' (p. 118). On the other hand, feelings of powerlessness were frequent. Powerlessness developed in health care settings through not being introduced to staff, staff's incompetence during procedures and depersonalisation (being treated like a 'lump of meat'). To regain control, one woman, Maree, insisted on being fully informed at all times and participating in decision making; she adopted specific strategies post-operatively:

> When she woke connected to a ventilator and a variety of invasive monitoring devices, she soon learned to remove the pulse meter from her finger which activated an alarm. Staff responded to this and once more she felt in control in the intensive care environment, an extremely controlling context for all patients. To establish equal control with the medical staff she always sat up and insisted on shaking their hands when they arrived at the bedside. This enabled her to gain level eye contact, which she perceived as reducing any potential power imbalance of either a patient/doctor or able bodied/disabled body nature.
>
> (Lumby 1997: 119)

Maree was labelled as difficult in health care settings, and she found that she was labelled as a 'liver transplant' in her work setting, which led to further feelings of disempowerment on returning to work. Lumby reports that Maree was able to link her fear of losing control and her fight for control to her family experiences, in which she felt easily 'put down by men'. Whereas her father and brothers were valued for their large physiques, she was, as a big woman, chastised for eating too much and felt ashamed of her body. She felt that her size had 'denigrated her as a female' (p. 120). For Maree, and for many women in the study, after surviving a transplant, 'because they had faced life and death and taken control, they were changed and determined to take control of their future in ways which their families did not always understand or accept' (Lumby 1997: 122). Women with the most traditional family role patterns found least acceptance for their changed, more confident identity. Perhaps as a result, many women found strong support from other women.

Lumby's work illustrates how women's experiences of their body and changes in their body through illness affect their enactment of gendered roles and often reinforce feelings of disempowerment through the vulnerability of being perceived as an inferior woman. The threats to identity and to roles, however, often lead to a reaffirmation of their strengths as women, such as their skills in organising and in emotional labour, developed through the need to employ their skills for personal survival and the wellbeing of others. Families are organised through careful planning in order to minimise disruption to their lives while the women themselves are hospitalised. Women use communication skills and emotional labour to find ways of controlling themselves and those responsible for their care. Nurses can seek to understand these strategies and support women in developing coping strategies and personal styles. Ensuring that a patient is sitting up, ready to talk to the doctor, is an example.

Disempowerment through taking power away is common in hospital settings despite the rhetoric of patients' choice and patients' rights. In other health care settings, disempowerment through an overt control over patients' lives can be part of the culture of an organisation. Lee-Treweek's (1998) analysis of the control that a nursing auxiliary has over 'bedroom work' in a nursing home illustrates the possibilities for controlling practices in personal care to become abusive. She found that although untrained staff viewed physical abuse towards patients as unacceptable, within the auxiliaries' 'subculture of personal hardship... acts of mistreatment and punishment were pervasive and unquestioned' (Lee-Treweek 1998: 235). The abuse was verbal; ignoring buzzers or individual needs was common. The verbal abuse was an important part of younger women's strategies in maintaining control over the older residents and over the stresses on themselves as carers. Lee-Treweek (1998) reports that the auxiliaries tolerated violence from patients on a daily basis.

Gender, violence and health care

Power exerted over another often takes the form of physical violence. The trauma experienced by individuals through violence can have long-term and severe consequences for social relationships and mental health. As Busfield (1996) notes, war is the ultimate exercise of power, and the emergence of 'shell-shock' as a disabling condition had an important place in the history of psychiatry and of the construction of masculinity. 'Shell-shock' came to be accepted as a psychiatric disorder after the experience of World War One, in which the number of cases and the fact that officers were apparently more affected than the lower ranks made it 'difficult to maintain that those who manifested the symptoms should be treated as cowards or malingerers and court-martialled' (p. 218). Its acceptance was significant 'in view of the harsh attitudes and strict values of the military and the threat shell-shock posed to military strength and morale, to conceptions of masculinity and to assumptions of male agency' (p. 218). As Busfield notes, this was one instance when it was fortuitous to be able to deny male agency and rationality; 'shell-shock' allowed the military to refute an alternative view – that men wished to ignore their duty to fight and felt fear in combat. Psychiatric services increased significantly between the wars, partly through the acceptance of neuroses among men. The term 'shell-shock' has, however, been replaced by the concept of 'post-traumatic stress disorder'. Although the DSM-IV (APA 1994) list includes rape as a traumatic event, it does not include domestic violence as 'trauma'.

Sexual violence (and linked factors)

Sexual violence is often traumatic and can have long-term consequences for survivors in terms of anxiety, anger, hostility, depression, changed attitudes towards men (who are usually the perpetrators), including a distrust of men, fear, hatred or anger (Busfield 1986). There is a high incidence of suicide attempts reported among those who have experienced sexual abuse as a child (Browne and Finkelhor 1986). Nevertheless, it is not helpful to overemphasise the negative consequences for individuals. Perpetuating the 'victim' status of survivors can reinforce the relative powerlessness that may have contributed to the abuse and can ignore and denigrate the strategies that individuals use for their own successful survival.

The experience of health care can, however, often be particularly difficult for the survivors of sexual abuse. Kitzinger (1997) found this to be the case in research with 40 women who were survivors of childhood (mainly incestuous) assaults. She notes that sexual abuse can affect women's views of their bodies, leading them to detest their own bodies, to feel alienated from their own sexual organs and to perceive physical examinations as intrusions that renew feelings of vulnerability. Vaginal examinations can lead to flashbacks in which a woman feels she is a child again, re-experiencing an assault. Others cope with examinations by 'switching off', and the 'rituals designed to desexualise encounters with health carers (such as lack of eye contact or the isolated focus on a woman's genitals) can actually make women feel depersonalised and treated "just like an object"' (Kitzinger 1997: 89). Some women may feel especially vulnerable in the presence of male staff. Understandably, childbirth can be a particularly difficult experience for women survivors of sexual abuse, and negative encounters with health care practitioners can make each subsequent contact with health services a significant ordeal. Kitzinger found that

> Some incest survivors may approach childbirth as if they are totally helpless; they may be utterly subservient and unable to express their own desires. Others regard the midwife as a potential assailant. They refuse to negotiate and insist on rigid rules about what the midwife can or cannot do. They react to any deviation from pre-agreed plans as if it is an immense betrayal of trust.

> (1997: 89)

Women's behaviour may make midwives or any health professional feel undermined by the evident lack of trust in their skills and professionalism, but an understanding of the reasons for women's responses can help professionals to find ways to ensure that women feel respected and in control. 'A gentle examination, a listening ear and a respectful approach can all help women to 'reclaim' their bodies' (p. 93). Kitzinger provides guidelines for midwives in caring for women survivors. These include being informed about sexual violence, being open to the possibility that women in their care have experienced abuse, respecting confidentiality and fears about disclosure, accepting pain, distress and negative views of health care and thinking about possible extra needs for support with breastfeeding. Reflecting on one's own attitudes and reactions to ensure that communication remains positive between all involved is important, and thinking through each aspect of practice from the standpoint of a women who has been sexually assaulted may help to develop and change practice.

Ferguson (1994) gives guidance for the care of women who are depressed, with a view to enhancing the nurse's ability to provide women with opportunities to disclose experiences of abuse. Nevertheless, disclosure remains the woman's choice, within her control. Questions might include open invitations to describe their lives and their feelings in general, particularly in relation to roles as a wife, a mother, a woman, for example 'what support do you have from other people?' Are there any changes you would like to make to your life? Do you feel able to make them? How are things with your partner? Tell me about things that have been happening recently. How do you feel about them? Tell me about your past life with your own family. Do you feel that any events from the past have influenced how you feel about yourself now?' (Ferguson 1994: 113). These are all questions that help nurses to demonstrate their willingness to listen. Further examples of mental health workers providing supportive services for women through a woman-centred approach have already been referred to in Chapters 9 and 10. Berry et al. (1993) have identified the importance of strong support and supervision systems to help nurses to deal with the feelings of helplessness and sadness that can arise through working with survivors of child sexual abuse.

Sheehan and Holley (1993) describe an innovative project providing support not just for the survivors of abuse, but also for the partners of the survivors of abuse. The facilitators of the partners' group were taken aback by the depth of emotional turmoil. Partners described feelings of outrage against abuse and the perpetrator and anger at themselves for not realising the extent of the women's distress, as well at themselves and others for failing to prevent it. There was an overwhelming sense of frustration, and widespread uncertainty about their own sexual and intimate behaviour. Sheehan and Holley (1993) term the women's partners' distress 'secondary sexual abuse' and note the widespread effects of disclosure and 'the hidden epidemic of fear, anger, guilt, frustration and confusion among the spouses, lovers and friends of women who have been sexually abused' (p. 22). Even more hidden is the effect of the abuse of men. The physical and sexual abuse of young men, often under the 'protection' of social and educational services, has only recently been made visible (Levy and Kahan 1991).

Physical abuse (and linked factors)

Pahl (1995) argues that health professionals fail to detect violence against women despite the fact that abused women are more likely to be in touch with the health service, particularly through general practitioners, than any other agency. Research in the United States has explored the effects of staff training in accident and emergency departments and the use of a protocol including questions to ask about the experience of abuse (McLeer and Anwar 1989). The results of the study showed that the identification of women who had experienced abuse increased from 5.6 per cent to 30 per cent through training and the use of the protocol. The researchers conclude that staff in accident and emergency departments should maintain a high degree of suspicion with regard to the prevalence of abuse and introduce protocols for the care of women attending with injuries. Protocols would identify the importance of accessible information concerning other services that could meet women's needs.

Pahl stressed that health professionals are well placed to help abused women, who seek help in different ways, including seeking a sympathetic listener and source of 'moral, medical or material support' (Pahl 1995: 132). Dobash et al. (1985) classified women's requests for help according to whether they were looking for support or for a challenge to the violence. Whereas the first request for help was more likely to be a request for support, requests for assistance to challenge the violence subsequently increased. Black women experience additional difficulties in challenging violence alongside racism (Mama 1989).

Pahl notes that health visitors are potentially an accessible source of help for abused women, but her own study, conducted twenty years ago, found that health visitors were not able to offer the expected help. Many of the women saw the health visitors as being concerned with the children rather than with themselves as mothers; others had tried to talk to the health visitors but felt that the response was inappropriate, the health visitor seeing the problem as the woman's or seeking a strategy 'for reconciliation when the wife was asking for support in challenging the violence' (Pahl 1995: 139). 'Some health visitors seemed to behave as though the wife had no claim to be helped in her own right, as though her welfare was subsumed under the heading of the welfare of the family or of the children' (p. 139). A further difficulty in gaining support from health visitors was their partners' suspicion of all visitors to the house.

On the basis of her research and her experience of educating health professionals, Pahl provides recommendations for good practice. These include respecting a woman's account of her experiences, having available relevant information concerning supportive local agencies, keeping careful records of any injuries and ensuring easy access to such information for the appropriate professionals, and giving enough time to women and their concerns. Health professionals whom the women had found supportive had organised their own work to meet the woman's needs, for example giving the last appointment of the day in a general practioner surgery, or calling at the house only when the husband's van was not outside to ensure that the discussions with the health visitor could be private.

Health care professionals have, however, made considerable progress in developing good practice in the care of abused women (Hadley 1992). Campbell and Humphreys (1993) provide a comprehensive guide for action, within a discussion of the context of violence against women, including machismo and patriarchy (Pahl 1995: 146). Jezierski (1992) has produced a protocol for intervention that includes suggestions for the phrasing of questions, a protection and safety plan and an emergency escape kit. Pahl (1995) reproduces this plan.

Men's violence to known women

Hearn (1998) identifies two differing emphases in explanations of men's violence to women, both influenced by psychoanalytic theory. One view sees violence as emerging from men's attempts to exert dominance through exaggerated masculinity, while the other sees violence as developing from an attempt to deny dependency and to hide femininity, again through dominance. Gilligan (1996), in an account of his knowledge gained through working with prison inmates as a psychiatrist, notes,

> I have yet to see a serious act of violence that was not provoked by the experience of feeling shamed and humiliated, disrespected and ridiculed, and that did not represent the attempt to prevent or undo this 'loss of face'.

> (p. 110)

Wilkinson *et al.* (1998) draw on Gilligan's work to emphasise the importance of crime and violence as public health issues, noting that 'Are you dis'in me?' (disrespecting me) is 'the standard way young people on the streets of Britain threaten belligerence' (p. 29). Hearn (1998) suggests that the overarching social context of men's violence is 'heteropatriarchal relations, structures and cultures'. In his research with men concerning their violence towards known women, he found that heteropatriarchal relations were ever-present yet implicit. The explicit accounts concerned employment, family situations, their past experiences in relationships with their parents, their own abuse, institutional living and a description of recent deterioration in their relationship with a woman through drink, depression and stress.

Hearn found that, in men's accounts of their own violence, women are 'strangely other and absent'. 'A *very limited, empty* portrayal of the woman is made' (Hearn 1998: 82). Men often described their violence as occasional rather than serious, as a reaction, and saw their real problems as lying elsewhere – in depression, addiction, upbringing, experience in care institutions. Men referred to the research project from different agencies defined their violence differently. Men involved with the police structured the events as exceptional, out of character; they were able to 'decentre' themselves in their accounts of the violence. Men referred from the probation service had a normalised and natu-ralised view of violence and did not focus on violence as an aspect of their behaviour in need of justification. Men in prison saw their violence as either the 'accident' of murder or incidental to their real criminality. Those who joined the research but were not referred from a statutory agency did not see their violence as a major theme in their lives. Hearn concluded that many agencies that have contact with men who are violent to known women do not necessarily focus on the violence:

> Intervention still rests largely on the woman being willing to convert a private conversation with a professional worker to a more public action outside the confines of the home. The private has to become public.
>
> (1998: 161)

Although the police response to domestic violence is changing, Hearn noted varied practices among the police services and the Crown Prosecution Service. The Probation Service appeared to demonstrate a lack of involvement in encouraging men to confront their violence, and social services worked more with the women involved rather than the men. Set in the context of Hearn's research, Pahl's comments on the inattention of health professionals suggest that agencies primarily involved with women and those primarily involved with men have all failed to focus sufficiently on violence and failed to work together to address men's violence to known women. Hearn recommends that all agencies should include more attention to the links between men's violence to known women, child protection work and support work with women. There is a need for a more focused recognition of men's violence and more focused work around this problem.

Hearn (1998) notes the importance of talking about violence in a collectivity in order to ensure that any collectivity, such as a work organisation, actively works against violence in thought, talk and deed. He notes the legitimising of violence within controlling organisations such as prisons and the police force. Hierarchical structures bring organisational values of power and domination, not ideal places to challenge a cultural acceptance of violence. Throughout his account of his research, Hearn demonstrates a reflexive sensitivity to the discourses he produces about violence in an attempt to describe the discourses produced by the men he interviewed. All explanations should be similarly examined in terms of the consequences of the accounts of behaviour for the perpetuation of that behaviour itself.

Interactionist explanations of violence, for example, would see the social world as being constructed through an interaction between self and other, through the reflexive capacity to 'take the role of the other'. In violence, as Hearn identified, the woman appeared to be 'other', but the man had no capacity to empathise with the other's standpoint. Many men perpetrating violence may see their own and women's roles in terms of rigid roles of domination and subordination, roles that have been seen as functional within certain social structures. Feminisms see such structures as patriarchal. More recently, feminisms have been criticised for casting women into too subordinate a victim role. Structuralist explanations can argue that 'capitalist relations of employment and unemployment might affect the gendered expectation and experiences of men and women, so that when men formerly defined as "breadwinners" become unemployed and identified as redundant they may reassert their selves through violence' (Hearn 1998: 207). Postmodernism suggests that discourses about men and women, about sexuality and about violence, can be reconstructed, but reconstructed through changing discourses that present men (and women) with the possibility that they have been wrong, not just in the sense of moral responsibility for an act, but also in the sense of being wrong in their view of the world. As Hearn (1998) notes, 'being wrong is very hard for most men to imagine. It is rare. It can be quite threatening to most men's sense of themselves, of what is usually called "identity"' (p. 199). Changing men's discourses about themselves might be more successfully accomplished if men's violence and women's abuse, as well as women's violence and men's abuse, could be addressed directly in agency and interagency work. Gender-sensitive care requires interagency support.

CONCLUSION

Gender, care and reciprocity

Nursing is a low-status profession in cultures that place value on economic success, on public leadership, on autonomy, on rationality and on theoretical knowledge. Gender is an issue for nursing because nursing's own devalued position is closely linked to women's status through the shared characteristics of the work that nurses and women do. Nursing involves caring through a responsiveness to others' actual or potential vulnerability and thus shares characteristics with mothering. 'The very nature of caring seems to be produced in the connection between the apparently ultimate vulnerability of early childhood and the potentially perfect responsiveness of mothers' (Bowden 1997: 21). Noddings (1984) and Ruddick (1989) have both used mothering to explore the characteristics of caring and caring relationships.

Women's caring, however, also involves care of the sick. Nursing as a profession can be seen to have developed from women's role in health and healing (Ehrenreich and English 1976). Women's work includes health work, and, within nursing, theorising nursing as health work has gained increasing importance, particularly since the Project 2000 educational reforms (UKCC 1986). Nursing has been characterised as emotional labour, involving a management of one's own and others' emotions that relies on, and cultivates, an awareness of interaction cues and a capacity for other-orientation that is associated with femininity rather than masculinity.

Nursing, like women's work, takes place in private settings. Nurses, like mothers, play a limited role in public organisations and in public policy, but for men and for women, it is public responsibilities that bring status and material rewards. Despite a sociological understanding of the links between private troubles and public issues (Mills 1970), men's and women's private troubles have little place in public activities. In public and professional activity, private troubles are seen as bringing with them an irrationality and emotionality that inhibit the impartial exercise of responsibility and distort decision making. Nevertheless, the skilled articulation of private troubles into public needs and the public representation of interests turns the irrational into the rational. Emotional awareness can lead to responsibility, partiality to the recognition of the importance of diversity, informal care into community care, personal health into public health, and nursing into policy for health and social care.

Women as providers, negotiators and mediators of health care

Feminist social science analyses have helped to identify gender issues in health and in health care. Explanations for women's higher rates of reporting of mental distress have centred on the difficulties of managing diverse demands on inadequate resources and on the negative effects of the physical demands and social isolation involved in caring responsibilities in the home (Payne 1991, Graham 1993).

Graham (1985) has provided an illuminating analysis of the processes involved in women's health care in the home, arguing that 1960s and 70s social science analyses of health care systems had, through an emphasis on health professions, ignored the processes of informal care. Graham (1985) describes women's roles in informal, unpaid work to protect and promote the health of others as those of provider, negotiator and mediator. Women's role as provider of health involves

> the provision of a materially-secure environment: a warm, clean home where both young and old can be protected against danger and disease, and a diet sufficient in quantity and quality to meet their nutritional needs. It involves, too, the provision of a social environment conducive to normal health and development.
>
> (p. 26)

The provision of a social environment conducive to health involves the development and transmission of a culture 'in which health and illness can be understood' (p. 26). Providing healthy food is not the same as ensuring that family members will eat it or choose such food for themselves.

Studies of lay referral systems (Zola 1973) illustrate the complexity of negotiating definitions of sickness and health, although they do not necessarily identify gender issues in the patterns of negotiation. As Graham (1985) argues, women are often key to such negotiation, yet through their role in the management of resources available to promote health, 'the burden of sacrifice falls not on others, but on the woman herself' (p. 39). Graham's research on women's smoking vividly illustrates this. Smoking provides a way of coping with unremitting demands through providing 'time out' for relaxation. It also serves, if necessary, as a substitute for food (Graham 1976).

Finally, women's role as negotiator involves mediation with formal care agencies. The wife-mother acts as gate-keeper between family and the outside world and has been traditionally relied upon by formal care agencies to mediate between private and public health systems. Graham (1985) notes that although the role of mediator suggests that there is a limit to the responsibilities of the private carer – as the responsibility for care can be handed over to professionals – it is the sense of responsibility that is the 'central motif in women's accounts of caring' (p. 36). Care in the community policies involve attempts at a reconfiguration of responsibility for care and support, attempts that were, as identified in Chapter 6, proclaimed in feminist scholarship as imposing new burdens on women. Gregor (1997) has argued that nurses should rethink their support for health policies supporting the expansion of primary health care. Since it is women who care in the home, such policies are not gender neutral; 'nurses themselves participate in conditions that snare and oppress women' (Gregor 1997: 35).

Graham's (1985) analysis, and Gregor's position, can be criti-cised for ignoring the complexity of gender relationships in informal care and the possibilities for a more radical restructuring of community services that will take gender issues seriously. Such restructuring could involve more community- (rather than indi-vidually) based responsibility for social support and health. However, the significance of Graham's argument that gender and privacy intersect to structure experience and identity through what Dahl and Snare (1978) have described as 'the coercion of privacy' should not be overlooked. The significance for nursing is that the privacy of their own care in private or in public settings also ensures that nurses' role as provider, negotiator and mediator of health care is hidden. The doctor–nurse game (Stein 1967) is a game of negotiation and mediation by a provider. Increasingly, as health care policy emphasises the importance of user participation and the centrality of primary and community care, professionals, as providers, are being encouraged to recognise the importance of their own responsibilities as negotiators and mediators. Davies' (1995) new model of professionalism could facilitate this. Analyses remain silent, however, on the importance of 'organising' as the hidden process that links provision with negotiation and mediation, practical tasks with communicative skills and emotional labour, and nursing 'work' with nursing 'care' (James 1992a, 1992b). In both public and private settings, 'lost is the daily reality of caring' (Graham 1985: 32). In Chapter 8, I suggest that this reality may be identified and revalued through making the importance of organising, and the negotiation involved in teamwork, clear in the public world of organisations.

Men and informal care

A closer examination of the daily reality of caring, in the private world as well as the public, has revealed that it is not only women who are enmeshed in the responsibilities of care. Just as social scientists have reconsidered the evidence relating to gender differences in morbidity (Macintyre *et al.* 1996, Arber 1997), a closer examination of informal care has revealed the extent and nature of men's participation (Arber and Gilbert 1989). The recognition of the role of men as informal caregivers derived initially from a concern to understand the experiences of older people and, more generally, from the broad recognition during the 1980s that initial feminist theorising in social science concentrated predominantly on the issues for younger and middle-aged, able-bodied, educated, middle-class, white women. As Rose and Bruce (1995) identify, a much more complex account of caring emerged in the 1990s, an account that drew on an understanding of differences, including cultural differences in the exploration of care relationships. Scandinavian research on care, for example, draws on relational aspects of care. Ve (1984) distinguished between three types of informal care: mutual care between equals, care necessary for survival, and personal servicing extracted through patriarchal relations of dominance. The Scandinavian tradition (Eliasson 1989, Simonen 1990) was also able to conceptualise paid carers not as agents of social control but as 'solidaristic towards the cared for' (Rose and Bruce 1995: 115). Within the Scandinavian literature, the rights of the cared-for could be considered along with the rights of the carers. The British concern for women's equal opportunities had curiously negated the rights of the cared-for through a concern to free women from the negative consequences of personal servicing care. Unsurprisingly, in British feminist social science literature, it has been the subordinated and exploitative nature of nursing personal service care that has been emphasised. Nurses' own attempts to articulate a sense of solidaristic concern for the rights of the cared-for have not necessarily been supported in social science literature on care.

Rose and Bruce (1995) note that 'the 1985 GHS findings that older male spouses did almost as much caring as older female spouses were received with considerable suspicion in feminist circles' (p. 116–17). The suspicion was articulated through critiquing the interpretation of the questions asked in the General Household Survey and the answers given (Green 1990). A question concerning 'extra family responsibilities', for example, cannot control for gender differences in assumptions about 'normal' family responsibilities. Nevertheless, Arber and Gilbert (1989) are clear that over one third of co-resident carers were men and that assumptions about men receiving more help from the voluntary and statutory services were not borne out by the data. Differences in the receipt of care were more related to the type of household and the presence of others in the household who could participate in care. Older people living alone received more help than those living with others. Married daughters caring for parents, however, received less support than unmarried carers, whether male or female. The majority of male carers were caring for a spouse or were single men caring for a parent. In such instances, the bonds are likely to be strong, and the relationship between carer and cared-for is likely to have changed, or to be changing, from one of reciprocity to one of dependence.

Rose and Bruce (1995) explored the nature of reciprocity and dependency through a postal questionnaire to 1,000 men and 1,000 women aged over 65, selecting, from the 989 returns, 16 couples for interview. In eight of the couples the man was more dependent, and in eight the woman was the dependent partner. The study revealed some gender differences that reflected a power imbalance between men and women; women were 'particularly vulnerable to denying themselves small pleasures because their husband is incapable of enjoying them as well' (Rose and Bruce 1995: 122), and wives felt more threatened by violent behaviour and personality changes resulting from strokes or dementia. Nevertheless, the study revealed a considerable flexibility of the gender division of tasks in order to 'maintain highly-valued independence as a couple' (p. 120). The language of care involved accounts of feelings of loss alongside a presentation of care activities as commonplace, a conversational strategy supporting a coping strategy that minimised the extreme difficulties.

Rose and Bruce (1995) explored issues concerning gender and coping, noting the complexity of the arguments surrounding connectedness, distance, caring and rationality. Bury and Holme (1991) found that a study of people aged over 90 suggested that men coped better than women with their caring responsibilities because they were more detached about the person they cared for. Such a view may contradict Gilligan's (1982) arguments about the importance of connectedness and care. Rose and Bruce found evidence of creative, controlled and confident caring by male carers, in which their care for their partner was salient with their self-perception as the protector of their wife. Caring could be seen as the continuation of their provider role. As interviewers, Rose and Bruce were puzzled by the ease with which they, as feminist researchers, could describe the men they interviewed as 'wonderful', whereas reproducing positive pictures of women as carers was more difficult for the interviewees and for the researchers. They comment,

> merely to attempt to care is admirable in a man, whereas for a woman it is her natural duty, and not only should she attempt it, but she feels under an obligation to perform well. The differential esteem felt by and for the older carer speaks eloquently of the long and deforming fingers of gender.
>
> (1995: 127–8)

Caring in later life

The importance of care relationships in later life for our understanding of the denigration of care and of gender relationships has not yet been fully explored. The valuing of men's and women's roles and activities rests on a differential value at different stages of the lifecourse. Functionalist, Marxist and feminist sociologies attest to the dominance of the economic and materialist necessity for labour that generates resources in determining the value system of a society. As such, the importance of 'provider' and paid employment activities to individuals, families, communities and societies affect individuals' financial rewards, status and class position. Financial provider status also affects the experience of dependence, independence, power and control. Women may be the providers of health and health care in the private sphere because they buy, cook and serve the food; but all those who provide financial support for a family group contribute to the materially secure environment that protects against danger and disease. Ignoring men's role in such provision is a feminist fiction that may have distorted our understanding of men's other-orientation and distorted our understanding of the pressures felt by men if they perceive themselves as failing in their protective role. If men in later life care with confidence, compassion and competence in organising their caring tasks, as well as managing their emotional labour, our analysis of gender relations may have been neglecting key features of responsibility, interdependence and reciprocity. Men's concern for others' welfare in the private sphere has been ignored.

The role of reciprocity and obligation in the 'daily reality of caring' has been explored by Neufeld and Harrison (1998). In a study of 22 male caregivers, 12 described their caring as being based on obligation rather than reciprocity. A sense of responsibility could be seen as a 'central motif' (Graham 1985) in men's accounts of caring. Among the 10 men who described feelings of reciprocity, the researchers identified three variations in reciprocity: waived reciprocity, generalised reciprocity and constructed reciprocity. Husbands with positive prior relationships with their wives were content to care for partners without any expectation of reciprocity. Generalised reciprocity involved an expectation that assistance would be returned by the family or community if necessary, but not by the cared-for individual. Such notions of reciprocity were part of a general altruistic value to contribute to the needs of others and of society. Constructed reciprocity involved individual attention to the detail of interaction and non-verbal behaviour through which a mutually caring relationship was constructed in the presence of communication difficulties associated with the cared-for's health. Some men described a transition from constructed reciprocity to caring by obligation. In comparison with a similar study of women's caring relationships, Neufeld and Harrison found that men were less likely than women to care on the basis of constructed reciprocity and more likely to move towards care through obligation. Men who used constructed reciprocity were less explicit than women in their descriptions of the interaction cues through which reciprocity was constructed.

Despite the limited nature of research concerning reciprocity, the lines of enquiry employed by Neufeld and Harrison suggest that men as well as women accept the obligations of care and that men may be more willing than women to accept the duty of care in the absence of a perception of reciprocity. However, more negative feelings about care were expressed by those caring through obligation than by those caring through reciprocity. Nursing assessment could include a discussion with carers concerning reciprocity and obligation, and a recognition that caring through obligation can be accompanied by negative or mixed feelings that may promote stress or depression could help to inform nursing interventions. Constructed reciprocity may, however, be facilitated by 'coaching in the observation of non verbal cues' (Neufeld and Harrison 1998: 967). Nurses' own care work could involve developing constructed reciprocity. In my experience as a nurse, I viewed carers' descriptions of their own interpretations of the cared-for's behaviour as an attempt to encourage nurses to provide individualised care for their partner, friend or relative.

It is possible that further explorations of gender differences in the ethical as well as the interpersonal basis of public and private caregiving, may enhance our understanding of gender and care. Men and women providing private care on the basis of assumptions about public duty as well as private obligations and affective relationships may be introducing elements of rational and impersonal responsibility into personal relationships that are in fact supportive of high standards of care. In caring relationships, universal values of autonomy, equity and justice can, and do, beneficially accompany particularities of individual concern. Nursing could contribute to an understanding of formal and informal care through articulating the relationship between public ethics and private practice. Neufeld and Harrison's (1998) interest in reciprocity and in men's informal care begins this process.

Kaye and Applegate (1995) describe three trends that they see as supportive of men's entry into the world of caregiving: younger fathers are increasingly playing an active role in childcare; demographic changes, including a lower birth rate, are resulting in a declining younger population relative to older people, increasing the possibility of adult children, both male and female, providing care for their parents in later life; and there is a growing recognition among employers of men's caring responsibilities. There are opportunities, therefore, for men 'to reconceptualise the meaning of gender' (Kaye and Applegate 1995: 218) through their caregiving. Nurses, both men and women, can participate in this process through their personal practice and through their own analyses of gender, health and care. Such analyses can not only take into account the negative consequences of powerful ideologies that construct restrictive masculinities and femininities, but also acknowledge reciprocity in care and gender relationships as well as the interdependence of public and private worlds, and of formal and informal care. Gender remains an issue for nursing, but health care is men's and women's work.

REFERENCES

Abbott P and Wallace C (1990) *An Introduction to Sociology: Feminist Perspectives*. Routledge, London.

Abbott P and Wallace C (1997) *An Introduction to Sociology: Feminist Perspectives*, 2nd edn. Routledge, London.

Abel-Smith B (1960) *A History of the Nursing Profession*. Heinemann, London.

Acheson D (1998) *Independent Inquiry into Inequalities in Health*. Stationery Office, London.

Acker J (1990) Hierarchies, jobs and bodies: a theory of gendered organisations. *Gender and Society* **4**: 139–58.

Adkins L (1995) *Gendered Work: Sexuality, Family and the Labour Market*. Open University Press, Milton Keynes.

Alderton J S (1991) The New Male Nurse. MSc dissertation in Social Research. University of Surrey and the Steinberg Collection, RCN, London.

Allan H T (1993) Feminism: a concept analysis. *Journal of Advanced Nursing* **18**: 1547–53.

American Psychiatric Association (1994) *Diagnostic and Statistical Manual of Mental Disorders*, 4th edn (DSM-IV). American Psychiatric Association, Washington.

Anderson J M, Dyck I and Lynam J (1997) Health care professionals and women speaking: constraints in everyday life and the management of chronic illness. *Health* **1**(1): 57–80.

Annandale E (1996) Working on the front-line: risk culture and nursing in the new NHS. *Sociological Review* **44**: 416–51.

Annandale E (1998a) Health Illness and the Politics of Gender. In Field D and Taylor S (eds) *Sociological Perspectives on Health Illness and Health Care*. Blackwell, Oxford, pp. 115–33.

Annandale E (1998b) *The Sociology of Health and Medicine: A Critical Introduction*. Polity Press, Cambridge.

Annandale E and Hunt K (1990) Masculinity, femininity and sex: an exploration of their relative contribution to explaining gender differences in health. *Sociology of Health and Illness* **12**: 24–46.

Arber S (1990) Opening the 'Black Box': Inequalities in Women's Health. In Abbott P and Payne G (eds) *New Directions in the Sociology of Health*. Falmer, Basingstoke, pp. 37–56.

Arber S (1997) Comparing inequalities in women's and men's health. *Social Science and Medicine* **13**(4): 199–201.

Arber S and Gilbert N (1989) Men: the forgotten carers. *Sociology* **23**(1): 111–18.

Arber S, Gilbert N and Dale A (1985) Paid employment and women's health: a benefit or a source of role strain? *Sociology of Health and Illness* 7: 375–99.

Armstrong D (1983) *Political Anatomy of the Body: Medical Knowledge in Britain in the Twentieth Century*. Cambridge, Cambridge University Press.

Ashley J A (1980) Power in structured misogyny: implications for the politics of care. *Advances in Nursing Science* 2(3): 3–22.

Atkinson J (1986) *Changing Work Patterns: How Companies Achieve Flexibility To Meet New Needs*. National Economic Development Office, London.

Austin R (1977) Sex and gender in the future of nursing. 1. *Nursing Times*, Occasional Paper, 73: 113–16.

Bachrach P and Baratz M S (1962) Two faces of power. *American Political Science Review* 56(4): 947–52.

Bakan D (1966) *The Duality of Human Existence*. Rand McNally, Chicago.

Baker D and Taylor H (1997) Inequality in health and health service use for mothers of young children in south west England. *Journal of Epidemiology and Community Health* 51: 74–9.

Balint M, Hunt J, Joyce D, Marinker M and Woodcock J (1970) *Treatment or Diagnosis: A Study of Repeat Prescriptions in General Practice*. Tavistock Publications, London.

Bandura A (1977) Self-efficacy: toward a unifying theory of behaviour change. *Psychological Review* 84: 191–215.

Barker D L and Allen S (eds) (1976) *Sexual Divisions and Society: Process and Change*. Macmillan, Basingstoke.

Barrett M (1980) *Women's Oppression Today*. Verso, London.

Bartley M (1994) Unemployment and ill health: understanding the relationship. *Journal of Epidemiology and Community Health* 48(4): 233–37.

Bartley M, Popay J and Plewis I (1992) Domestic conditions, paid employment and women's experience of ill-health. *Sociology of Health and Illness* 14: 314–43.

Beemer B R (1996) Gender dysphoria update. *Journal of Psychosocial Nursing* 34(4): 12–19.

Bellaby P and Oribabor P (1980) 'The History of the Present' – Contradiction and Struggle in Nursing. In Davies C (ed.) *Rewriting Nursing History*. Croom Helm, London, pp. 147–74.

Bem S L (1974) The measurement of psychological androgyny. *Journal of Consulting and Clinical Psychology* 42: 155–62.

Benner P (1984) *From Novice to Expert: Excellence and Power in Clinical Nursing*. Addison-Wesley, Menlo Park, CA.

Benner P and Wrubel J (1989) *The Primacy of Caring*. Addison-Wesley, London.

Berger J (1972) *Ways of Seeing*. Penguin, Harmondsworth.

Berry D, Drury J, Ranganathan P and Sumner J (1993) Sexual abuse: giving support to nurses. *Nursing Standard* 8(4): 25–7.

Bewley C (1999) Postnatal depression. *Nursing Standard* 13(16): 49–54.

Bhavnani K-K and Phoenix P (eds) (1994) *Shifting Identities, Shifting Racisms – a Feminism and Psychology Reader*. Sage, London.

Billington R, Hockey J and Strawbridge S (1998) *Exploring Self and Society*. Macmillan, Basingstoke.

Blaxter M (1990) *Health and Lifestyles*. Tavistock-Routledge, London.

Blazer D (1982) Social support and mortality in an elderly community population. *American Journal of Epidemiology* 115: 684–94.

Bloor M and McIntosh J (1990) Surveillance and Concealment: A Comparison of Techniques of Client Resistance in Therapeutic Communities and Health Visiting. In Cunningham Burley S and McKeganey N (eds) *Readings in Medical Sociology*. Routledge, London, pp. 159–81.

Bordo S (1990) Reading the Slender Body. In Jacobus M, Keller E F and Shuttleworth S (eds) *Body Politics: Women and the Discourse of Science*. Routledge, London, pp. 83–112.

Botting B (1997) Mortality in Childhood. In Drever F and Whitehead M (eds) *Health Inequalities: Decennial Supplement*: DS Series, No. 15. Stationery Office, London.

Bourdieu P (1986) *Distinction*. Routledge, London.

Bowden P (1997) *Caring: Gender-Sensitive Ethics*. Routledge, London.

Bowlby J (1953) *Child Care and the Growth of Love*. Penguin, London.

Brannon R (1976) The Male Sex Role: Our Culture's Blueprint of Manhood, and What It's Done for Us Lately. In Brannon D D and Brannon R (eds) *The Forty Nine Percent Majority*. Addison-Wesley, Reading, MA, pp. 1–45.

Brannon R and Juni S (1984) A scale for measuring attitudes about masculinity. *Psychological Documents* 14(1): ms. 2612.

Briggs A (1972) *Report of the Committee on Nursing*. Chairman Asa Briggs, Cmnd 5115. London, HMSO.

Brittain V (1978) *Testament of Youth*. Virago, London.

Brockbank W (1970) *History of Nursing at Manchester Royal Infirmary*. Manchester, Manchester University Press.

Brooks F and Phillips D (1996) Do women want women health workers? Women's views of the primary health care service. *Journal of Advanced Nursing* 23: 1207–11.

Broom L and Selznick P (1973) *Sociology*, 5th edn. Harper & Row, New York.

Broverman I K, Broverman D M, Clarkson F E, Rosenkrantz P S and Vogel S R (1970) Sex-role stereotypes and clinical judgments of mental health. *Journal of Consulting and Clinical Psychology* 34: 1–7.

Brown G and Harris T (1978) *The Social Origins of Depression*. Tavistock, London.

Brown R G S and Stones R W H (1970) Men who come into nursing. 1. *Nursing Times*, Occasional Paper. October 15: 153–55.

Browne A and Finkelhor D (1986) Impact of child sexual abuse: a review of research. *Psychological Bulletin* 99: 66–77.

Bruch H (1973) *Eating Disorders: Obesity, Anorexia and the Person Within*. Basic Books, New York.

Bruch H (1978) *The Golden Cage: The Enigma of Anorexia Nervosa*. Vintage, New York.

Buchan J, Seccombe I and Smith G (1998) *Nurses Work: An Analysis of the UK Nursing Labour Market*. Developments in Nursing and Health Care 18. Ashgate, Aldershot.

Burstow B (1992) *Radical Feminist Therapy: Working in the Context of Violence*. Sage, London.

Bury M (1982) Chronic illness as biographical disruption. *Sociology of Health and Illness* 4(2): 167–82.

Bury M (1991) The sociology of chronic illness: a review of research and prospects. *Sociology of Health and Illness* 8(2): 137–69.

Bury M (1997) *Health and Illness in a Changing Society*. Routledge, London.

Bury M and Holme A (1991) *Life After Ninety*. Routledge, London.

Busfield J (1996) *Men, Women and Madness*. Macmillan, Basingstoke.

Butler J (1993) *Bodies that Matter: On the Discursive Limits of 'Sex'*. Routledge, London.

Cameron E and Bernades J (1998) Gender and Disadvantage in Health: Men's Health for a Change. In Bartley M, Blane D and Davey Smith G (eds) *The Sociology of Health Inequalities*. Blackwell, Oxford, pp. 115–34.

Campbell J C and Bunting S (1991) Voices and paradigms: perspectives on critical and feminist theory in nursing. *Advances in Nursing Science* 13(3): 1–15.

Campbell J and Humphreys J (1993) *Nursing Care of Survivors of Family Violence*. Mosby, London.

Canaan J E (1996) 'One Thing Leads to Another': Drinking, Fighting and Working-class Masculinities. In Mac an Ghaill M (ed.) *Understanding Masculinities*. Open University Press, Buckingham, pp. 114–25.

Canetto S (1992–93) She died for love and he for glory: gender myths of suicidal behaviour. *Omega* 26: 1–17.

Canetto S (1995) Men Who Survive a Suicidal Act. In Sabo D and Gordon D F (eds) *Men's Health and Illness: Gender, Power and the Body*. Sage, London, pp. 292–304.

Carpenter M (1980) Asylum Nursing Before 1914: A Chapter in the History of Labour. In Davies C (ed.) *Rewriting Nursing History*. Croom Helm, London, p. 123–46.

Carpenter M (1993) The Subordination of Nurses in Health Care: Towards a Social Divisions Approach. In Riska E and Wegar K (eds) *Gender, Work and Medicine*. Sage, London, pp. 95–130.

Champagne J (1996) Homo Academicus. In Smith P (ed.) *Boys: Masculinities in Contemporary Culture*. West View Press, Oxford, pp. 49–79.

Charles J and Curtis L (1994) Birth afterthoughts – a listening and information service. *British Journal of Midwifery* 2: 331–4.

Charles N and Walters V (1998) Age and gender in women's accounts of their health. *Sociology of Health and Illness* **20**(3): 330–50.

Charmaz K (1991) *Good Days, Bad Days: The Self in Chronic Illness and Time*. Rutgers University Press, New Brunswick, NJ.

Charmaz K (1995) Identity Dilemmas of Chronically Ill Men. In Sabo D and Gordon D F (eds) *Men's Health and Illness: Gender, Power and the Body*. Sage, London, pp. 266–91.

Chesler P (1972) *Women and Madness*. Doubleday, New York.

Chinoy E (1967) *Society*, 2nd edn. Random House, New York.

Chodorow N (1978) *The Reproduction of Mothering*. University of California Press, Berkeley, CA.

Cixous H (1980) The Laugh of the Medusa, trans. K. Cohen and P. Cohen. In Marks E and de Courtivron I (eds) *New French Feminisms*. Harvester, Brighton, pp. 90–9.

Cixous H (1986) Sorties. In Cixous H and Clement C *The Newly Born Woman*. Manchester University Press, Manchester.

Clark D C (1993) Narcissistic crises of aging and suicidal despair. *Suicide and Life Threatening Behaviour* **23**: 21–6.

Clark J Macleod (1993) From Sick Nursing to Health Nursing: Evolution or Revolution. In Wilson-Barnett J and Clark J Macleod (eds) *Research in Health Promotion and Nursing*. Macmillan, Basingstoke, pp. 256–70.

Clark P (1997) Male order problems. *Nursing Times* **93**(10): 32–3.

Collins P Hill (1990) *Black Feminist Thought: Knowledge, Consciousness and the Politics of Empowerment*. HarperCollins, London.

Collinson D L and Hearn J (eds) (1996) *Men as Managers, Managers as Men*. Sage, London.

Colyer H (1996) Women's experience of living with cancer. *Journal of Advanced Nursing* **23**: 496–501.

Connell R W (1987) *Gender and Power*. Polity Press, Cambridge.

Connell R W (1993) The big picture: masculinities in recent world history. *Theory and Society* **22**: 597–624.

Connell R W (1995) *Masculinities*. Polity Press, Cambridge.

Connell R W, Ashenden D J, Kessler S and Dowsett G W (1982) *Making the Difference*. Allen & Unwin, Sydney.

Cook E P (1985) *Psychological Androgyny*. Pergamon Press, USA.

Cornwall A and Lindisfarne N (eds) (1994) *Dislocating Masculinity: Comparative Ethnographies*. Routledge, London.

Cowan P J (1996) Women's mental health issues: reflections on past attitudes and present practices. *Journal of Psychosocial Nursing* **34**(4): 20–4.

Coyle J (1999) Exploring the meaning of 'dissatisfaction' with health care: the importance of 'personal identity threat'. *Sociology of Health and Illness* **21**(1): 95–124.

Cribb A and Dines A (1993) What is Health Promotion? In Dines A and Cribb A (eds) *Health Promotion: Concepts and Practice*. Blackwell Scientific Publications, Oxford, pp. 20–32.

Dahl T and Snare A (1978) The Coercion of Privacy: A Feminist Perspective. In Smart C and Smart B (eds) *Women, Sexuality and Social Control*. Routledge & Kegan Paul, London.

Dalley G (1988) *Ideologies of Caring: Rethinking Community and Collectivism*. Macmillan, London.

Dally A (1982) *Inventing Motherhood: The Consequences of an Ideal*. Burnett Books, London.

Dalton K (1985) Progesterone prophylaxis used successfully in postnatal depression. *Practitioner* **229**: 507–8.

Daly M (1979) *Gyn/Ecology: The Meta-Ethics of Radical Feminism*. Women's Press, London.

Davies C (ed.) (1980) *Rewriting Nursing History*. Croom Helm, London.

Davies C (1992) Gender, History and Management Style in Nursing: Towards a Theoretical Synthesis. In Savage M and Witz A (eds) *Gender and Bureaucracy*. Blackwell, Oxford.

Davies C (1995) *Gender and the Professional Predicament in Nursing*. Open University Press, Buckingham.

Davies C and Rosser J (1986) *Processes of Discrimination: A Study of Women Working in the NHS*. DHSS/HMSO, London.

Davis M A (1981) Sex differences in reporting osteoarthritis symptoms: a sociomedical approach. *Journal of Health and Social Behaviour* **22**: 298–310.

Delphy C (1977) *The Main Enemy*. Women's Research and Resource Centre, London.

Department of Health (1989a) *Caring for People: Community Care in the Next Decade and Beyond*. HMSO, London.

Department of Health (1989b) *Working for Patients*. HMSO, London.

Department of Health (1997) *The New NHS: Modern, Dependable*. Stationery Office, London.

Department of Health (1998a) *Our Healthier Nation*. Stationery Office, London.

Department of Health (1998b) *Supporting Families*. Stationery Office, London.

Department of Social Security (1997) *Social Security 1997 Statistics*. Stationery Office, London.

Dingwall R, Rafferty A M, Webster C (1988) *An Introduction to the Social History of Nursing*. Routledge, London.

Dobash R E, Dobash R P and Cavanagh K (1985) The Contact Between Battered Women and Social and Medical Agencies. In Pahl J (ed.) *Private Violence and Public Policy*. Routledge and Kegan Paul, London, pp. 142–65.

Dolan B (1990) Project 2000, the gender mender? *Nursing Standard* **4**(47): 52–3.

Dominelli L (1997) *Sociology for Social Work*. Macmillan, Basingstoke.

Donald J (1985) Beacons of the Future: Schooling, Subjection and Subjectification. In Beechey V and Donald J (eds) *Subjectivity and Social Relations*. Open University Press, Milton Keynes.

Doyal L (1987) Infertility – A Life Sentence? Women and the National Health Service. In Stanworth M (ed.) *Reproductive Technologies: Gender, Motherhood and Medicine*. Polity Press, Cambridge, pp. 174–90.

Doyal L (1995) *What Makes Women Sick? Gender and the Political Economy of Health*. Macmillan, Basingstoke.

Drever F and Bunting J (1997) Patterns and Trends in Male Mortality. In Drever F and Whitehead M (eds) *Health Inequalities: Decennial Supplement*: DS Series No. 15. Stationery Office, London, pp. 95–107.

Dunnell K (1991) Deaths among 15–44 year olds. *Population Trends* **64**: 38–43.

Edwards A (1989) The sex/gender distinction – has it outlived its usefulness? *Australian Feminist Studies* **10**: 1–12.

Egeland J and Brown J (1988) Sex role stereotyping and role strain of male registered nurses. *Research in Nursing and Health* **11**(4): 257–67.

Ehrenreich B and English D (1976) *Witches, Midwives and Nurses: A History of Women Healers*. Writers and Readers Publishing Cooperative, London.

Eisler R M and Skidmore J R (1987) Masculine gender role stress: scale development and component factors in the appraisal of stressful situations. *Behaviour Modification* **11**(2): 123–36.

Eisler R M, Skidmore J R and Ward C H (1988) Masculine gender-role stress: predictor of anger, anxiety, and health-risk behaviours. *Journal of Personality Assessment*, **52**:133–41.

Eisner M and Wright M (1986) A Feminist Approach to General Practice. In Webb C (ed.) *Feminist Practice in Women's Health Care*. John Wiley & Sons, Chichester, pp. 113–45.

Eliasson R (1989) Perspectives and Outlooks in Social Science Research. In Elzinga A (ed.) *In Science We Trust?* Lund University Press, Lund.

Ellerby K (1988) A career in nursing. *Nursing Times* **84**(8): 59–61.

Engels F (1985 [1884]) *The Origin of the Family, Private Property and the State*. Penguin, Harmondsworth.

Epstein D (1996) Keeping Them in Their Place: Hetero/Sexist Harassment, Gender and the Enforcement of Heterosexuality. In Holland J and Adkins L (eds) *Sex, Sensibility and the Gendered Body*. Macmillan, Basingstoke, pp. 202–21.

Etzioni A (1969) *The Semi-professions and their Organisations*. Free Press, New York.

Evandrou M (1996) Unpaid Work, Carers and Health. In Blane D, Brunner E and Wilkinson R (eds) *Health and Social Organisation*. Routledge, London, pp. 204–31.

Evans J (1997) Men in nursing: issues of gender segregation and hidden advantage. *Journal of Advanced Nursing* **26**: 226–31.

Farnworth M (1952) The social prestige of nursing. *Nursing Times*, June 21: pp. 684–5.

Farr K A (1988) Dominance bonding through the good old boys sociability group. *Sex Roles* **18**(5/6): 259–78.

Ferguson K (1994) Mental Health and Sexuality. In Webb C (ed.) *Living Sexuality: Issues for Nursing and Health*. Scutari Press, London, pp. 99–119.

Few C (1997) The politics of sex research and constructions of female sexuality: what relevance to sexual health work with young women? *Journal of Advanced Nursing* **25**: 615–25.

Finch J (1990) The Politics of Community Care in Britain. In Ungerson C (ed.) *Gender and Caring: Work and Welfare in Britain and Scandinavia*. Harvester Wheatsheaf, Hemel Hempstead.

Finch J and Groves D (eds) (1983) *A Labour of Love: Women, Work and Caring*. Routledge & Kegan Paul, London.

Firestone S (1979) *The Dialectic of Sex: The Case for Feminist Revolution*. Women's Press, London.

Fleming V E M (1998) Women and midwives in partnership: a problematic relationship? *Journal of Advanced Nursing* **27**: 8–14.

Foster P (1989) Improving the doctor–patient relationship: a feminist perspective. *Journal of Social Policy* **18**(3): 337–61.

Foucault M (1980) Power/Knowledge. In Gordon C (ed. and trans.) *Selected Interviews and Other Writings*. Harvester Wheatsheaf, Brighton.

Fox N (1993) *Postmodernism, Sociology and Health*. Open University Press, Buckingham.

Fox N (1995) Postmodern perspectives on care: the vigil and the gift. *Critical Social Policy* **44/45**: 107–25.

Franks P and Clancy C M (1993) Physician gender bias in clinical decision making: screening for cancer in primary care. *Medical Care* **31**: 213–18.

Frazier F (1966) *The Negro Family in the United States*. University of Chicago Press, Chicago.

Freud S (1973) Femininity. In *New Introductory Lectures on Psychoanalysis*. Penguin, Harmondsworth.

Freud S (1977) *On Sexuality*. Pelican Freud Library, Vol. 7. Penguin, Harmondsworth.

Freud S (1984) *On Metapsychology: The Theory of Psychoanalysis*. Pelican Freud Library, Vol. 11. Penguin, Harmondsworth.

Friedan B (1963) *The Feminine Mystique*. Norton, New York.

Gamarnikow E (1978) Sexual Division of Labour: The Case of Nursing. In Kuhn A and Wolpe A-M (eds) *Feminism and Materialism*. Routledge & Kegan Paul, London, pp. 96–123.

Geertz C (1993) *The Interpretation of Cultures*. Fontana, London (first published 1973).

Giddens A (1991) *Modernity and Self Identity*. Polity Press, Cambridge.

Gilligan C (1982) *In a Different Voice*. Harvard University Press, Cambridge, MA.

Gilligan J (1996) *Violence: Our Deadly Epidemic and its Causes*. G P Putman, New York.

Gilloran A (1995) Gender differences in care delivery and supervisory relationship: the case of psychogeriatric nursing. *Journal of Advanced Nursing* 21: 652–8.

Gilmore D (1993) *Manhood in the Making. Cultural Concepts of Masculinity*. Yale University Press, New Haven, CT.

Godfrey J (1999) Empowerment Through Sexuality. In Wilkinson G and Miers M (eds) *Power and Nursing Practice*. Macmillan, Basingstoke, pp. 172–86.

Goffman E (1968) *Stigma: Notes on Management of Spoiled Identity*. Penguin, Harmondsworth.

Goffman E (1969) *The Presentation of Self in Everyday Life*. Penguin, Harmondsworth.

Goleman D (1998) *Working with Emotional Intelligence*. Bloomsbury, London.

Gordon D F (1995) Testicular Cancer and Masculinity. In Sabo D and Gordon D F (eds) *Men's Health and Illness: Gender, Power and the Body*. Sage, London, pp. 246–65.

Gordon M (1998) Empowerment and Breastfeeding. In Kendall S (ed.) *Health and Empowerment*. Edward Arnold, London, pp 154–84.

Gordon R A (1990) *Anorexia and Bulimia: Anatomy of a Social Epidemic*. Blackwell, Oxford.

Gove W R and Tudor J F (1973) Adult sex roles, mental illness and marital status. *Social Forces* 51(1): 34–44.

Graham H (1976) Smoking in pregnancy: attitudes of expectant mothers. *Social Science and Medicine* 10: 399–405.

Graham H (1983) Caring: A Labour of Love. In Finch J and Groves D (eds) *A Labour of Love: Women, Work and Caring*. Routledge & Kegan Paul, London.

Graham H (1985) Providers, Negotiators, and Mediators: Women as the Hidden Carers. In Lewin E and Oelsen V (eds) *Women, Health and Healing: Toward a New Perspective*. Tavistock, London, pp. 25–52.

Graham H (1987) Women's smoking and family health. *Social Science and Medicine* 25(1): 47–56.

Graham H (1993) *Hardship and Health in Women's Lives*. Harvester Wheatsheaf, Brighton.

Gramsci A (1971) *Selections from the Prison Notebooks*. Lawrence & Wishart, London.

Green H (1990) Survey of carers: methodological problems. *Survey Methodology Bulletin* 26: 17–25. OPCS/HMSO, London.

Greene J (1992/3) Men in nursing and the Royal College of Nursing. *History of Nursing Journal* 4: 3–8.

Gregoire A J P, Kumar R, Everitt B, Henderson A F and Studd J W W (1996) Transdermal oestrogen for the treatment of severe postnatal depression. *Lancet* 347: 930–3.

Gregor F (1997) From women to women: nurses, informal caregivers and the gender dimension of health care reform in Canada. *Health and Social Care in the Community* 5(1): 30–6.

Greipp M E (1996) Client age, gender, behaviour: effects on quality of predicted self reactions and colleague reactions. *Nursing Ethics* **3**(2): 126–39.

Grimwood C and Popplestone R (1993) *Women, Management and Care*. Macmillan, Basingstoke.

Hadley S (1992) Working with battered women in the emergency department: a model programme. *Journal of Emergency Nursing* **18**(1): 18–23.

Hagell E I (1989) Nursing knowledge: women's knowledge. A sociological perspective. *Journal of Advanced Nursing* **14**: 226–33.

Halford S, Savage M and Witz A (1997) *Gender, Careers and Organisations*. Macmillan, Basingstoke.

Hallam J (1998) From angels to handmaidens: changing constructions of nursing's public image in post-war Britain. *Nursing Inquiry* **5**: 32–42.

Hammersley M (1992) On feminist methodology. *Sociology* **26**: 187–206.

Hannam J (1997) Women, History and Protest. In Robinson V and Richardson D (eds) *Introducing Women's Studies*, 2nd edn. Macmillan, Basingstoke, pp. 77–97.

Hargreaves J (1994) *Sporting Females*. Routledge, London.

Hearn J (1992) *Men in the Public Eye: The Construction and Deconstruction of Public Men and Public Masculinities*. Routledge, London.

Hearn J (1998) *The Violences of Men*. Sage, London.

Heinrich K T and Witt B (1993) The passionate connection: feminism invigorates the teaching of nursing. *Nursing Outlook* **41**: 117–24.

Helgeson V (1995) Masculinity, Men's Roles and CHD. In Sabo D and Gordon D F (eds) *Men's Health and Illness: Gender, Power and the Body*. Sage, California, pp. 68–104.

Henderson V (1966) *The Nature of Nursing*. Collier-Macmillan, London.

Hochschild A (1983) *The Managed Heart: Commercialisation of Human Feeling*. University of California Press, Berkeley, CA.

Holden J (1990) Emotional Problems Associated with Childbirth. In Alexander J, Levy V and Roch S (eds) *Midwifery Practice: Postnatal Care – A Research Based Approach*. Macmillan, London, pp. 45–61.

Holden J (1994) Using the Edinburgh Postnatal Depression Scale in Clinical Practice. In Cox J L and Holden J M (eds) *Perinatal Psychiatry: Use and Misuse of the EPDS*. Gaskell, London.

Holland S (1996) Developing a Bridge to Women's Social Action. In Heller T, Reynolds J, Gomm R, Muston R and Pattison S (eds) *Mental Health Matters*. Macmillan/Open University, Basingstoke, pp. 304–8.

Holloway W (1996) Masters and Men in the Transition from Factory Hands to Sentimental Workers. In Collinson D L and Hearn J (eds) *Men as Managers, Managers as Men*. Sage, London, pp. 25–42.

Holmes P (1987) Boy's talk. *Nursing Times* **87**(7): 29–31.

Holt R (1989) *Sport and the British*. Oxford University Press, Oxford.

hooks b (1991) *Yearning: Race, Gender and Cultural Politics*. Turnaround, London.

Horrocks R (1994) *Masculinity in Crisis*. Macmillan, Basingstoke.

House J S, Robbins C and Metzner H L (1982) The association of social relationships and activities with mortality: prospective evidence from the Tecumseh Community Health Study. *American Journal of Epidemiology* **116**: 123–40.

House of Commons (1904) *Report from the Select Committee on Registration of Nurses*. HMSO, London.

Hughes D (1988) When nurse knows best: some aspects of nurse/doctor interaction in a casualty department. *Sociology of Health and Illness* **10**: 1–22.

Hutt R (1985) *Chief Officer Career Profiles: A Study of the Backgrounds, Training and Career Experiences of Regional and District Officers*. Report No. 111. University of Sussex: Institute of Manpower Studies.

Ireland J (1993) Undoing Gender Segregation? A Comparison of Men in Nursing and Women in the Engineering Trades. Paper presented at National Study Day on Gender at Work, University of Luton, November 16th 1993.

James N (1989) Emotional labour: skill and work in the regulation of feelings. *Sociological Review* **37**: 15–41.

James N (1992a) Care = organisation + physical labour + emotional labour. *Sociology of Health and Illness* **14**(4):488–509.

James N (1992b) Care, Work and Carework: A Synthesis? In Robinson J, Gray A and Elkan R (eds) *Policy Issues in Nursing*. Open University Press, Buckingham, pp. 96–111.

Jezierski M (1992) Guidelines for intervention by ED nurses in cases of domestic abuse. *Journal of Emergency Nursing* **18**(1):298–300.

Johnson M (1994) Conflict and Nursing Professionalization. In McCloskey J and Grace H (eds) *Current Issues in Nursing*. Mosby, Toronto, pp. 643–9.

Jones L and Webb C (1994) Young Men's Experiences of Testicular Cancer. In Webb C (ed.) *Living Sexuality: Issues for Nursing and Health*. Scutari Press, London, pp. 32–49.

Jones M (1984) An Investigation into Attitudes Towards Men in Nursing with Particular Emphasis on Female Patient Care. BSc in Nursing Studies Dissertation. Polytechnic of the South Bank, London.

Kalisch P A and Kalisch B J (1982a) The image of the nurse on prime-time television. *American Journal of Nursing*, February: 265–70.

Kalisch P A and Kalisch B J (1982b) The image of the nurse in motion pictures. *American Journal of Nursing* April: 605–11.

Kanter R (1977) Some effects of proportions on group life: skewed sex ratios and responses to token women. *American Journal of Sociology* **82**(5): 965–90.

Kanter R M (1993) *Men and Women of the Corporation*. Basic Books, New York.

Kauppinen-Toropainen K and Lammi J (1993) Men in Female Dominated Occupations. A Cross Cultural Comparison. In Williams C (ed.) *Doing 'Women's Work'. Men in Nontraditional Occupations*. Sage, London, pp. 91–112.

Kaye L W and Applegate J S (1995) Men's Style of Nurturing Elders. In Sabo D and Gordon D F (eds) *Men's Health and Illness: Gender, Power and the Body*. Sage, London, pp. 205–21.

Keddy B C (1995) Feminist teaching and the older nurse: the journey from resistance through anger to hope. *Journal of Advanced Nursing* **21**: 690–4.

Kelleher D (1988) *Diabetes*. Routledge, London.

Kendall S (ed.) (1998) *Health and Empowerment: Research and Practice*. Edward Arnold, London.

Kendall-Thackett K A and Kaufman-Kanter G (1993) *Postpartum Depression: A Comprehensive Approach for Nurses*. Sage, London.

Kenny T (1991) Anorexia nervosa – a nursing challenge that can bring results. *Professional Nurse*, August: 666–9.

Kerfoot D and Knights K (1996) 'The Best is Yet to Come?': The Quest for Embodiment in Managerial Work. In Collinson D L and Hearn J (eds) *Men as Managers, Managers as Men*. Sage, London, pp. 78–98.

Kintz L (1996) Conservative Cowboy Stories: Adventures of the Chosen Sons. In Smith P (ed.) *Boys: Masculinities in Contemporary Culture*. Westview Press, Oxford, pp. 219–54.

Kirkham M (1986) A Feminist Perspective on Midwifery. In Webb C (ed.) *Feminist Practice in Women's Health Care*. John Wiley & Sons, Chichester, pp. 35–49.

Kitzinger J (1997) Sexual Violence and Midwifery Practice. In Kargar I and Hunt S C (eds) *Challenges in Midwifery Care*. Macmillan, Basingstoke, pp. 87–98.

Kitzinger S D (1992) Birth and Violence Against Women: Generating Hypotheses from Women's Accounts of Unhappiness after Childbirth. In Roberts H (ed.) *Women's Health Matters*. Routledge, London, pp. 63–80.

Klaus M H and Kennell J H (1976) *Maternal–Infant Bonding*. Mosby, St Louis.

Klein M (1946) Notes on some schizoid mechanisms. *International Journal of Psycho-Analysis* **27**: 99–110.

Komarovsky M (1946) Cultural Contradictions and Sex Roles. *American Journal of Sociology*, November.

Kondo D K (1990) *Crafting Selves: Power, Gender and Discourses of Identity*. University of Chicago Press, London.

Kuhse H (1997) *Caring: Nurses, Women and Ethics*. Blackwell, Oxford.

Lask S (1987) Beliefs and behaviour in health education. *Nursing* **3**: 681–3.

Latter S (1998) Health Promotion in the Acute Setting: The Case for Empowering Nurses. In Kendall S (ed.) *Health and Empowerment: Research and Practice*. Edward Arnold, London, pp. 11–37.

Lawler J (1991) *Behind the Screens: Nursing, Somology and the Problem of the Body*. Churchill Livingstone, Edinburgh.

Lawler J (ed.) (1997) *The Body in Nursing*. Churchill Livingstone, Melbourne.

Lawrence M (1987) Education and Identity: The Social Origins of Anorexia. In Lawrence M (ed.) *Fed Up and Hungry: Women, Oppression and Food*. Women's Press, London.

Lee Treweek G (1996) Emotion Work, Order, and Emotional Power in Care Assistant Work. In James V and Gabe J (eds) *Health and the Sociology of Emotions*. Blackwell, Oxford, pp. 115–32.

Lee Treweek G (1998) Bedroom Abuse: The Hidden Work in a Nursing Home. In Allott M and Robb M (eds) *Understanding Health and Social Care: An Introductory Reader*. Sage, London, pp. 230–5.

Lees S (1986) *Losing Out: Sexuality and Adolescent Girls*. Penguin, London.

Lees S (1993) *Sugar and Spice: Sexuality and Adolescent Girls*. Penguin, London.

Levy A and Kahan B (1991) *The Pindown Experience and the Protection of Children: The Report of the Staffordshire Child Care Inquiry 1990*. Staffordshire County Council, Stafford.

Lewis J and Meredith B (1988) *Daughters Who Care: Daughters Caring for Mothers at Home*. Routledge, London.

Lister R (1992) *Women's Economic Dependency and Social Security*. Equal Opportunities Commission, Manchester.

Lister R (1997) *Citizenship: Feminist Perspectives*. Macmillan, Basingstoke.

Littlewood J and McHugh N (1997) *Maternal Distress and Postnatal Depression: The Myth of Madonna*. Macmillan, Basingstoke.

Lloyd W A (1965) The male administrator. *Nursing Times*, March 12: 363–4.

Loden M (1985) *Feminine Leader: How To Succeed in Business Without Being One of the Boys*. Times Books, London.

Lodge N, Mallet J, Blake P and Fryatt I (1997) A study to ascertain gynaecological patients' perceived levels of embarrassment with physical and psychological care given by female and male nurses. *Journal of Advanced Nursing* 25: 893–907.

Long C G and Hollin C R (1995) Assessment and management of eating disordered patients who over-exercise: a four year follow-up of six single case studies. *Journal of Mental Health* 4(3): 309–16.

Lorber J (1997) *Gender and the Social Construction of Illness*. Sage, California.

Luker K A, Beaver K, Leinster S J and Owens R G (1993) Preferences for Information and Decision Making in Women Newly Diagnosed with Breast Cancer: Final Report. Unpublished Report for the Cancer Relief Macmillan Fund, London.

Luker K A, Beaver K, Leinster S J and Owens R G (1996) Information needs and sources of information for women with breast cancer: a follow-up study. *Journal of Advanced Nursing* 23: 487–95.

Lukes S (1974) *Power: A Radical View*. Macmillan, Basingstoke.

Lumby J (1997) The Feminised Body in Illness. In Lawler J (ed.) *The Body in Nursing*. Churchill Livingstone, Edinburgh, pp. 109–33.

Mac an Ghaill M (1994) *The Making of Men: Masculinities, Sexualities and Schooling*. Open University Press, Buckingham.

Mac an Ghaill M (ed.) (1996) *Understanding Masculinities*. Open University Press, Buckingham.

MacDougall G (1997) Caring – a masculine perspective. *Journal of Advanced Nursing* **25**: 809–13.

McGown A and Whitbread J (1996) Out of control! The most effective way to help the binge-eating patient. *Journal of Psychosocial Nursing* **34**(1): 30–7.

McIntosh J (1993) Post partum depression: women's help seeking behaviour and perceptions of cause. *Journal of Advanced Nursing* **18**: 178–84.

Macintyre S (1976) Who Wants Babies? The Social Construction of Instincts. In Barker D L and Allen S (eds) *Sexual Divisions and Society: Process and Change*. Tavistock, London, pp. 150–73.

Macintyre S (1993) Gender differences in the perceptions of common cold symptoms. *Social Science and Medicine* **23**: 393–415.

Macintyre S and West P (1993) What does the phrase 'safer sex' mean to you? *AIDS* **7**(1): 121–5.

Macintyre S, Hunt K and Sweeting H (1996) Gender differences in health: are things as simple as they seem? *Social Science and Medicine* **32**(4): 395–402.

Mackay L (1989) *Nursing a Problem*. Open University Press, Buckingham.

Mackay L (1993) *Conflicts in Care: Medicine and Nursing*. Chapman & Hall, London.

Mackay L (1995) The Patient as Pawn in Interprofessional Relationships. In Soothill K, Mackay L and Webb C (eds) *Interprofessional Relations in Health Care*. Edward Arnold, London, pp. 349–60.

McKie L (1996) Women Hearing Men: The Cervical Smear Test and the Social Construction of Sexuality. In Holland J and Adkins L (eds) *Sex, Sensibility and the Gendered Body*. Macmillan, Basingstoke, pp. 120–35.

McLeer S and Anwar R (1989) A study of battered women presenting in an emergency department. *American Journal of Public Health* **79**(1): 65–6.

Maggs C (1980) Nurse Recruitment to Four Provincial Hospitals 1881–1921. In Davies C (ed.) *Rewriting Nursing History*. Croom Helm, London, pp. 18–40.

Maggs C (1986) Sarah Gamp's Daughters: The English Nurse in Fiction. Paper presented to Nursing and Anthropology Workshop, Oxford, April 26/27.

Mama A (1989) *The Hidden Struggle: Statutory and Voluntary Sector Responses to Violence Against Black Women in the Home*. Runnymede Trust, London.

Marmot M and Feeney A (1996) Work and Health: Implications for Individuals and Society. In Blane D, Brunner E and Wilkinson R (eds) *Health and Social Organisation*. Routledge, London, pp. 235–54.

Marsland L, Robinson S and Murrells T (1996) Pursuing a career in nursing: differences between men and women qualifying as general nurses. *Journal of Nursing Management* **4**(4): 231–41.

Mead G H (1934) *Mind, Self and Society.* University of Chicago Press, Chicago.

Meltzer H, Gill B, Petticrew M and Hinds K (1995) *The Prevalence of Psychiatric Morbidity Among Adults Living in Private Households.* Office of Population Censuses and Surveys/HMSO, London.

Menzies I (1970) *The Functioning of Social Systems as a Defense Against Anxiety.* Tavistock, London.

Mercer K and Julien I (1988) Race, Sexual Politics and Black Masculinity: A Dossier. In Chapman R and Rutherford J (eds) *Male Order: Unwrapping Masculinity.* Lawrence & Wishart, London, pp. 97–164.

Messner M (1990) When bodies are weapons: masculinity and violence in sport. *International Review for the Sociology of Sport* **25**(3): 203–18.

Middleton S (1987) Streaming and the Politics of Female Sexuality: Case Studies in the Schooling of Girls. In Weiner G and Arnot M (eds) *Gender Under Scrutiny: New Inquiries in Education.* Unwin Hyman, London, pp. 77–89.

Miers M (1979) Health Costs of Lifestyle. In Atkinson P, Dingwall R and Murcott A (eds) *Prospects for the National Health.* Croom Helm, London, pp. 102–17.

Miers M (1996) Do They Mean Us? *Nursing Standard* **10**(15): 20–1.

Miers M (1999a) Nurses in the Labour Market: Exploring and Explaining Nurses' Work. In Wilkinson G and Miers M (eds) *Power and Nursing Practice.* Macmillan, Basingstoke, pp. 83–96.

Miers M (1999b) Involving Clients in Decision Making: Breast Care Nursing. In Wilkinson G and Miers M (eds) *Power and Nursing Practice.* Macmillan, Basingstoke, pp. 187–203.

Miles A (1991) *Women, Health and Medicine.* Open University Press, Buckingham.

Millett K (1972) *Sexual Politics.* Abacus, London.

Milligan F (1993) *A Comprehensive Review of British Literature on Men in Nursing.* Faculty of Health Care and Social Studies, University of Luton, Luton.

Mills C Wright (1970) *The Sociological Imagination.* Penguin, Harmondsworth.

Ministry of Health and Scottish Home and Health Department (1966) *Report of the Committee on Senior Nursing Staff Structure.* Chairman, Brian Salmon. HMSO, London.

Minuchin S, Rosman B L and Baker L (1979) *Psychosomatic Families: Anorexia Nervosa in Context.* Harvard University Press, Massachusetts.

Moore J (1988) *A Zeal for Responsibility: The Struggle for Professional Nursing in Victorian England, 1868–1883.* University of Georgia Press, Atlanta.

Morris J (1993) *Independent Lives?: Community Care and Disabled People.* Macmillan, London.

Murray M and Chambers M (1990) Characteristics of students entering different forms of nurse training. *Journal of Advanced Nursing* **15**: 1099–105.

Murray R and Heulskoetter M (1983) *Psychiatric/Mental Health Nursing – Giving Emotional Care*. Prentice Hall, Englewood Cliffs, NJ.

Myrdal A and Klein V (1968) *Women's Two Roles,* 2nd edn. Routledge, London.

Neufeld A and Harrison M J (1998) Men as caregivers: reciprocal relationships or obligation? *Journal of Advanced Nursing* **28**(5): 959–68.

Newton L H (1981) In defence of the traditional nurse. *Nursing Outlook* **29**: 348–54.

Nicolson P (1986) Developing a Feminist Approach to Depression Following Childbirth. In Wilkinson S (ed.) *Feminist Social Psychology*. Open University Press, Milton Keynes.

Nicolson P (1997) Motherhood and Women's Lives. In Robinson V and Richardson D (eds) *Introducing Women's Studies*, 2nd edn. Macmillan, Basingstoke, pp. 375–99.

Nightingale F (1970 [1859]) *Notes on Nursing*. Duckworth, London.

Noddings N (1984) *Caring: A Feminine Approach to Ethics and Moral Education*. University of California Press, Berkeley, CA.

Nolan M and Grant G (1992) *Regular Respite: An Evaluation of a Hospital Rota Bed Scheme for Elderly People*. Research Monograph Series, Age Concern Institute of Gerontology. ACE Books, London.

Nolan P (1989) Attendant dangers. *Nursing Times* **85**(12): 56–9.

Nuttall P (1983) Male takeover or female give-away? *Nursing Times* **79**: 10–11.

Oakley A (1972) *Sex, Gender and Society*. Temple Smith, London.

Oakley A (1974) *The Sociology of Housework*. Martin Robertson, London.

Oakley A (1976) The Family, Marriage and its Relationship to Illness. In Tuckett D (ed.) *An Introduction to Medical Sociology*. Tavistock, London, pp. 74–109.

Oakley A (1979) *Becoming a Mother*. Martin Robertson, Oxford.

Oakley A (1993) On the Importance of Being a Nurse. In Oakley A, *Essays on Women, Medicine and Health*. Edinburgh University Press, Edinburgh, pp. 38–51.

Oakley A (1998) Gender, methodology and people's ways of knowing: some problems with feminism and the paradigm debate in social science. *Sociology* **32**(4): 707–31.

Oates M (1988) The Development of an Integrated Community Orientated Service for Severe Postnatal Depression. In Kumar R and Brockington I E (eds) *Motherhood and Mental Illness* 2. Wright, London, pp. 133–58.

Office for National Statistics (1997) *Smoking in Secondary School Children*. Stationery Office, London.

Office for National Statistics (1998a) *Mortality Statistics: Cause 1996*. Series DH2, No. 23. Stationery Office, London.

Office for National Statistics (1998b) *1992 Cancer Statistics: Registrations*. Series MB1, No. 25. Stationery Office, London.

Office for National Statistics (1999) *Social Trends No. 29*. Stationery Office, London.

Orbach S (1993) *Hunger Strike*, 2nd edn. Penguin, Harmondsworth.

Orbach S (1998 [1978]) *Fat is a Feminist Issue*, I and II. Arrow Books, London.

Ozga J (ed.) (1993) *Women in Educational Management*. Open University Press, Buckingham.

Pahl J (1995) Health Professionals and Violence Against Women. In Kingston P and Penhale B (eds) *Family Violence and the Caring Professions*. Macmillan, Basingstoke, pp. 127–48.

Parker G (1990) *With Due Care and Attention: A Review of Research on Informal Care*, 2nd edn. Family Policy Studies Centre, London.

Parkin W (1989) Private Experiences in the Public Domain: Sexuality and Residential Care Organisations. In Hearn J, Sheppard D L, Tancred-Sheriff P and Burrell G (eds) *The Sexuality of Organisations*. Sage, London, pp. 110–24.

Parrish J (1962) Top level training of women in the U.S., 1900–1960. *Journal of the Association of Women Deans and Counsellors*, January.

Parsons T (1951) *The Social System*. Free Press, New York.

Parsons T and Bales R F (1953) *Family, Socialisation and Interaction Process*. Routledge & Kegan Paul, London.

Payne S (1991) *Women, Health and Poverty: An Introduction*. Harvester Wheatsheaf, Brighton.

Pearson A (1988) *Primary Nursing: Nursing in Burford and Oxford Development Units*. Croom Helm, Beckenham.

Pennebaker J W, Kiecolt-Glaser J K and Glaser R (1988) Disclosure of traumas and immune function: health implications for psychotherapy. *Journal of Consulting and Clinical Psychology* 56: 239–45.

Perry P (1993) From HMI to Polytechnic Director. In Ozga J (ed.) *Women in Educational Management*. Open University Press, Buckingham, pp. 82–96.

Phoenix A (1991) *Young Mothers?* Polity Press, London.

Piani A and Schoenborn C (1993) *Health promotion and disease prevention, United States, 1990*. Vital and Health Statistics, Series 10, No. 185. DHHS Pub No. 93–1513. Department of Health and Human Services, Hyattsville, MD.

Piper S (1997) The limitations of well men clinics for health education. *Nursing Standard* 11(30): 47–9.

Pleck J H, Sonenstein F L and Ku L C (1993) Masculinity Ideology and its Correlates. In Oskamp S and Costanzo M (eds) *Gender Issues in Contemporary Society*. Sage, Newbury Park, CA, pp. 85–110.

Plumwood V (1989) Do we need a sex/gender distinction? *Radical Philosophy* 51: 2–11.

Porter S (1992) Women in a women's job: the gendered experience of nurses. *Sociology of Health and Illness* 14: 510–27.

Porter S (1998) *Social Theory and Nursing Practice*. Macmillan, Basingstoke.

Porter S (1999) Working with Doctors. In Wilkinson G and Miers M (eds) *Power and Nursing Practice*. Macmillan, Basingstoke, pp. 97–110.

Pringle M Kellmer (1980) *A Fairer Future for Children*. Macmillan, Basingstoke.

Pringle R (1989) *Secretaries Talk: Sexuality, Power and Work.* Verso, London.

Pronger B (1990) *The Arena of Masculinity, Sports, Homosexuality and the Meaning of Sex.* St Martin's Press, New York.

Purves L (1997) Lads know best. *Nursing Standard* 11(23): 19.

Ramazonoglu C (1992) On feminist methodology: male reason versus female empowerment. *Sociology* 26: 207–12.

Ratcliffe P (1996) Gender differences in career progress in nursing: towards a non-essential structural theory. *Journal of Advanced Nursing* 23(2): 389–95.

Reverby S (1987a) *Ordered to Care: The Dilemma of American Nursing, 1850–1945.* Cambridge University Press, Cambridge.

Reverby S (1987b) A caring dilemma: womanhood and nursing in historical perspective. *Nursing Research* 36: 5–11.

Richardson D (1993) *Women, Motherhood and Childrearing.* Macmillan, Basingstoke.

Rhodes P (1994) *Nice Girls Don't Do That. Gender, Pollution and Professional Boundaries in the Performance of Intimate Procedures for Patients with Continence Problems.* British Sociological Association Annual Conference on Sexualities in Social Context, Preston, March.

Roberts H (1985) *The Patient Patients: Women and their Doctors.* Pandora, London.

Roberts S (1983) Oppressed group behaviour: implications for nurses. *Advances in Nursing Science* 5(4): 21–30.

Robinson I (1988) *Multiple Sclerosis.* Routledge, London.

Robinson V and Richardson D (eds) (1997) *Introducing Women's Studies,* 2nd edn. Macmillan, Basingstoke.

Rodwell C (1996) An analysis of the concept of empowerment. *Journal of Advanced Nursing* 23: 305–13.

Romans P (1992) Daring to Pretend? Motherhood and Lesbianism. In Plummer K (ed.) *Modern Homosexualities.* Routledge, London, pp. 98–107.

Rose H and Bruce E (1995) Mutual Care but Differential Esteem: Caring Between Older Couples. In Arber S and Ginn J (eds) *Connecting Gender and Ageing: A Sociological Approach.* Open University Press, Buckingham, pp. 114–28.

Rosen J G and Jones K (1972) The male nurse. *New Society,* March 9: 493–4.

Rousseau J (1966) *Emile* (trans. B Foxley). Dent, London.

Ruddick S (1989) *Maternal Thinking: Toward a Politics of Peace.* Beacon Press, Boston.

Russell G F M (1977) The present status of anorexia nervosa. *Psychological Medicine* 7: 353.

Ryan S and Porter S (1993) Men in nursing: a cautionary comparative critique. *Nursing Outlook* 41(6): 262–7.

Sabo D and Gordon D F (1995) Rethinking Men's Health and Illness. In Sabo D and Gordon D F (eds) *Men's Health and Illness: Gender, Power and the Body.* Sage, London, pp. 1–21.

Salvage J (1992) The New Nursing: Empowering Patients or Empowering Nurses? In Robinson J , Gray A and Elkan R (eds) *Policy Issues in Nursing*. Open University Press, Buckingham, pp. 9–23.

Savage J (1995) *Nursing Intimacy*. Scutari Press, Harrow.

Savage M and Witz A (1992) *Gender and Bureaucracy*. Blackwell, Oxford.

Segal L (1997) Feminist Sexual Politics and the Heterosexual Predicament. In Segal L (ed.) *New Sexual Agendas*. Macmillan, Basingstoke, pp. 77–89.

Seidler V (1988) Fathering, Authority and Masculinity. In Chapman R and Rutherford J (eds) *Male Order: Unwrapping Masculinity*. Lawrence & Wishart, London, pp. 272–302.

Shajahan P M and Cavanagh J T O (1998) Admission for depression among men in Scotland, 1980–95: retrospective study. *British Medical Journal* **316**: 1496–7.

Sharp K (1994) Sociology and the nursing curriculum: a note of caution. *Journal of Advanced Nursing* **20**: 391–5.

Sheehan A and Holley C (1993) Secondary sexual abuse. *Nursing Standard* **8**(4): 22–3.

Simonen L (1990) Caring by the Welfare State and the Women Behind it: Contradictions and Theoretical Considerations. In Simonen L (ed.) *Finnish Debates on Women's Studies*. University of Tampere, Tampere.

Simson M (1953) Is nursing a vocation? *Nursing Times*, September 5: p. 899.

Skeggs B (1986) Young Women and Further Education: A Case Study of Young Women's Experience of Caring Courses in a Local College. Unpublished PhD dissertation. University of Keele, Keele.

Skeggs B (1997) *Formations of Class and Gender*. Sage, London.

Sloan G (1999) Anorexia nervosa: a cognitive behavioural approach. *Nursing Standard* **13**(19): 143–7.

Smart C (1996) Desperately Seeking Post-Heterosexual Woman. In Holland J and Adkins L (eds) *Sex, Sensibility and the Gendered Body*. Macmillan, Basingstoke, pp. 222–41.

Smith P (1992) *The Emotional Labour of Nursing*. Macmillan, Basingstoke.

Smith P (ed.) (1996) *Boys: Masculinities in Contemporary Culture*. Westview Press, Oxford.

Sofer C (1955) Reactions to administrative change: a study of staff relationships in three British hospitals. *Human Relations* **8**: 291–316.

Spence J, Brackx A and Margolis L (1978) Facing Up to Myself. *Spare Rib* **68**: 6–9.

Spence J T, Helmreich R L and Stapp J (1974) The personal attributes questionnaire: a measure of sex-role stereotypes and masculinity-femininity. *JSAS Catalogue of Selected Documents in Psychology* **4**: 127.

Stacey J (1997) Feminist Theory: Capital F, Capital T. In Robinson V and Richardson D (eds) *Introducing Women's Studies*, 2nd edn. Macmillan, Basingstoke, pp. 54–76.

Stanley L (ed.) (1990) *Feminist Praxis: Research, Theory and Epistemology in Feminist Sociology*. Routledge, London.

Stanworth M (1987) *Reproductive Technologies: Gender, Motherhood and Medicine*. Polity Press, Cambridge.

Staples R (1982) *Black Masculinity: The Black Male's Role in American Society*. New Beacon Books, London.

Stein L (1967) The doctor–nurse game. *Archives of General Psychiatry* **16**: 699–703.

Stein L, Watts D T and Howell T (1990) The doctor–nurse game revisited. *New England Journal of Medicine* **322**: 546–9.

Stillion J M (1995) Premature Death Among Males. In Sabo D and Gordon D F (eds) *Men's Health and Illness: Gender, Power and the Body*. Sage, Newbury Park, CA, pp. 46–67.

Sturt J (1998) Implementing Theory into Primary Health Care Practice: An Empowering Approach. In Kendall S (ed.) *Health and Empowerment: Research and Practice*. Edward Arnold, London, pp. 38–56.

Stryker S (1962) Conditions of Accurate Role-Taking: A Test of Mead's Theory. In Rose A M (ed.) *Human Behaviour and Social Processes: An Interactionist Approach*. Routledge & Kegan Paul, London, pp. 41–62.

Sullivan A (1995) *Virtually Normal: An Argument About Homosexuality*. Macmillan, Basingstoke.

Summers A (1988) *Angels and Citizens: British Women as Military Nurses 1854–1914*. Routledge & Kegan Paul, London.

Summers A (1989) Pride and Prejudice: Ladies and Nurses in the Crimean War. In Samuel R (ed) *Patriotism: The Making and Unmaking of British National Identity*. Vol. II: *Minorities and Outsiders*. Routledge, London, pp. 57–78.

Symonds A and Hunt S (1996) *The Midwife and Society: Perspectives, Policies and Practice*. Macmillan, Basingstoke.

Tait A (1990) The Mastectomy Experience. In Stanley L (ed.) *Feminist Praxis*. Routledge, London, pp. 172–88.

Taylor B M (1995) Gender-power relations and safer sex negotiation. *Journal of Advanced Nursing* **22**: 687–93.

Taylor F W (1947) *Scientific Management*. Harper & Row, New York.

Tewksbury R (1995) Sexual Adaptations Among Gay Men With HIV. In Sabo D and Gordon D F (eds) *Men's Health and Illness: Gender, Power and the Body*. Sage, London, pp. 222–45.

Tickle L (1996) Mortality trends in the United Kingdom, 1982–1992. *Population Trends* **86**: 21–8.

Tiefer L (1997) Medicine, Morality and the Public Management of Sexual Matters. In Segal L (ed.) *New Sexual Agendas*. Macmillan, Basingstoke, pp. 103–12.

Tilt E (1852) *Elements of Health and Principles of Female Hygiene*. London.

Tones K (1998) Health Education and the Promotion of Health: Seeking Wisely to Empower. In Kendall S (ed.) *Health and Empowerment: Research and Practice*. Edward Arnold, London, pp. 57–88.

Trobst K, Collins R L and Embree J M (1994) The role of emotion in social support provision: gender, empathy and expressions of distress. *Journal of Social and Personal Relationships* **11**: 45–62.

Twomey M (1986) A Feminist Perspective in District Nursing. In Webb C (ed.) *Feminist Practice in Women's Health Care*. John Wiley & Sons, Chichester, pp. 51–67.

Ungerson C (1987) *Policy is Personal: Sex, Gender and Informal Care*. Tavistock, London.

Ungerson C· (1997) Women and Informal Care: Introduction. In Ungerson C and Kember M (eds) *Women and Social Policy*. Macmillan, Basingstoke, pp. 343–6.

United Kingdom Central Council for Nursing, Midwifery and Health Visiting (1986) *Project 2000: A New Preparation for Practice*. UKCC, London.

United Kingdom Central Council for Nursing, Midwifery and Health Visiting (1992) *Scope of Professional Practice*. UKCC, London.

Ussher J (1991) *Women's Madness: Misogyny or Mental Illness*. Harvester Wheatsheaf, London.

Valentine P E B (1988) A Hospital School of Nursing: A Case Study of a Predominantly Female Organisation. Unpublished doctoral dissertation. University of Alberta, Edmonton.

Valentine P (1992) Feminism: a four letter word. *Canadian Nurse* December: 20–23.

Valentine P E B (1995) Management of conflict: do nurses/women handle it differently? *Journal of Advanced Nursing* **22**: 142–9.

Vandemeer Y G, Loendersloot E W and Van Loenen A C (1984) Effect of high dose progesterone in post partum depression. *Journal of Psychosomatic Obstetrics and Gynaecology* **3**: 67–8.

Ve H (1984) Women's Mutual Alliances: Altruism as a Basis for Interaction. In Holter H (ed.) *Patriarchy in a Welfare Society*. University of Bergen, Bergen.

Villeneuve M (1994) Recruiting and retaining men in nursing: a review of the literature. *Journal of Professional Nursing* **10**(4): 217–28.

Walby S (1990) *Theorising Patriarchy*. Basil Blackwell, Oxford.

Walby S, Greenwell J, Mackay L and Soothill K (1994) *Medicine and Nursing: Professions in a Changing Health Service*. Sage, London.

Waldron I (1995) Contributions of Changing Gender Differences in Behaviour and Social Roles to Changing Gender Differences in Mortality. In Sabo D and Gordon D F (eds) *Men's Health and Illness: Gender, Power and the Body*. Sage, Newbury Park, CA, pp. 22–45.

Walters E and Whitehead L (1997) Anorexia nervosa in a young boy with gender identity disorder. *Clinical Psychology in Psychiatry* **2**(3): 463–7.

Walters V, French S, Eyles J, Lenton R, Newbold B and Mayr J (1997) The effects of paid and unpaid work on nurses' well-being: the importance of gender. *Sociology of Health and Illness* **19**(3): 328–47.

Wardhaugh J and Wilding P (1993) Towards an explanation of the corruption of care. *Critical Social Policy* **37**: 4–31.

Watson J (1979) *The Philosophy and Science of Caring*. Little, Brown, Boston.

Watson J (1985) *Nursing: Human Science and Human Care: A Theory of Nursing*. Appleton-Century-Crofts, New York.

Webb C (1986) Women as Gynaecology Patients and Nurses. In Webb C (ed.) *Feminist Practice in Women's Health Care*. John Wiley & Sons, Chichester, pp. 93–112.

Webb C and Wilson Barnett J (1983) Coping with hysterectomy. *Journal of Advanced Nursing* **8**(3): 311–19.

Webb D (1998) A 'revenge' on modern times: notes on traumatic brain injury. *Sociology* **32**(3): 541–55.

Weber M (1948) *From Max Weber: Essays in Sociology* (ed. and trans. H H Gerth and C Wright Mills). Routledge & Kegan Paul, London.

Weeks J (1991) *Against Nature: Essays on History, Sexuality and Identity*. Rivers Oram Press, London.

Wenger N K (1994) Coronary heart disease in women: gender differences in diagnostic evaluation. *Journal of the American Medical Women's Association* **49**: 181–5.

Wheeler C E and Chinn P L (1991) *Peace and Power: A Handbook of Feminist Process*, 3rd edn. National League for Nursing Press, New York.

White H and Stillion J M (1988) Sex differences in attitudes towards suicide: do males stigmatise males? *Psychology of Women Quarterly* **12**: 357–72.

White J H (1991) Feminism, eating and mental health. *Advances in Nursing Science* **13**(3): 68–80.

White J and Schroeder M A (1986) Femininity, image, feminism and a decision to seek treatment in obese women. *Health Care Women International* **7**(6): 455–67.

White P G, Young K and McTeer W G (1995) Sport, Masculinity and the Injured Body. In Sabo D and Gordon D F (eds) *Men's Health and Illness: Gender, Power and the Body*. Sage, London, pp. 158–82.

White R (1985) *The Effects of the NHS on the Nursing Profession 1948–1961*. King Edward's Hospital Fund for London, London.

Whitley B E (1984) Sex role orientation and psychological well-being: two meta analyses. *Sex Roles* **12**: 207–25.

Whitton A, Warner R and Appleby L (1996) The pathway to care in postnatal depression: women's attitudes to postnatal depression and its treatment. *MIDIRS Midwifery Digest* **7**(1): 93–4.

Wilkinson G and Miers M (1999) Power and Professions. In Wilkinson G and Miers M (eds) *Power and Nursing Practice*. Macmillan, Basingstoke, pp. 24–36.

Wilkinson R G, Kawachi I and Kennedy B (1998) Mortality, the Social Environment, Crime and Violence. In Bartley M, Blane D and Davey Smith G (eds) *The Sociology of Health Inequalities*. Blackwell, Oxford, pp. 19–37.

Williams C L (1989) *Gender Differences at Work: Women and Men in Non-Traditional Occupations*. University of California Press, Los Angeles.

Williams C (1994) Nurses' Voices – Men in Nursing: Lazy? On the Glass Escalator? Or Gay? Conference paper: British Sociological Association Annual Conference, Sexualities in Social Context, March 28–31, University of Central Lancashire, Preston.

Williams G, Fitzpatrick R, MacGregor A and Rigby A S (1996) Rheumatoid Arthritis. In Davey B and Seale C (eds) *Experiencing and Explaining Disease*. Open University Press, Buckingham, pp. 27–52.

Williams J and Watson G (1996) Mental Health Services that Empower Women. In Heller T, Reynolds J, Gomm R, Muston R and Pattison S (eds) *Mental Health Matters*. Macmillan/Open University, Basingstoke, pp. 242–51.

Williams S J (1993) *Chronic Respiratory Disorder*. Routledge, London.

Willis P (1977) *Learning to Labour: How Working Class Kids Get Working Class Jobs*. Columbia University Press, New York.

Wilton T (1996) Which One's the Man? The Heterosexualisation of Lesbian Sex. In Richardson D (ed.) *Theorising Heterosexuality*. Open University Press, Buckingham, pp. 125–42.

Wilton T (1997) *En/gendering AIDS: Deconstructing Sex, Texts, Epidemic*. Sage, London.

Winship J (1983) Femininity and Women's Magazines: A Case Study of Woman's Own. Unit 6, Open University Course U221, *The Changing Experience of Women*. Open University Press, Milton Keynes.

Wittgenstein L (1958) *Philosophical Investigations*, 2nd edn. (trans. G E M Anscombe). Blackwell, Oxford.

Wittig M (1979) One is not born a woman. In *Proceedings of the Second Sex Conference*. Institute of the Humanities, New York.

Wittig M (1992) *The Straight Mind and Other Essays*. Harvester Wheatsheaf, Brighton.

Witz A (1992) *Professions and Patriarchy*. Routledge, London.

Wollstonecraft M (1970 [1792]) *A Vindication of the Rights of Women*. Dent, London.

Woodward J (1974) *To Do the Sick no Harm: A Study of the British Hospital System to 1875*. Routledge & Kegan Paul, London.

Worsley P (ed.) (1970) *Introducing Sociology*, 2nd edn. Penguin Books, Harmondsworth.

York University Students Union (1997) *Uncensored: Alternative Prospectus 1997–99 Entry*. York University Students Union, York.

Young E H and Lee R M (1996) Fieldworker Feelings as Data: 'Emotion Work' and 'Feeling Rules' in First Person Accounts of Sociological Fieldwork. In James V and Gabe J (eds) *Health and the Sociology of Emotions*. Blackwell, Oxford. pp. 97–113.

Zaretsky E (1976) *Capitalism, the Family and Personal Life*. Pluto, London.

Zola I (1973) Pathways to the doctor: from person to patient. *Social Science and Medicine* 7: 677–89.

Name Index

A

Abel-Smith B, 37, 71, 80
Abbott P, 7–8, 22, 24, 162
Acheson D, 49–50, 56–7, 187
Acker J, 150
Adkins L, 15, 150
Alderton J S, 107
Allan H T, 166
Allen S, 7
American Psychiatric
    Association, 209
Anderson J M, 197
Annandale E, 52–3, 55, 57–60,
    141
Anwar R, 212
Appelgate J S, 225
Arber S, 54–5, 123, 220–1
Armstrong D, 112
Ashley J A, 165
Association of Workers in
    Asylums, 89
Atkinson J, 155
Austin R, 104

B

Bachrach P, 201
Bakan D, 10
Baker D, 57
Bales R F, 18
Balint M, 54
Bandura A, 141
Baratz M S, 201
Barker D L, 7
Barrett M, 23
Bartley M, 54–5
Bedford Fenwick (Mrs), 86–8
Beemer B R, 179, 184
Bellaby P, 82–3
Bem S L, 59
Benner P, 112–13, 118–20,
    125, 198
Berger J, 35

Bernades J, 63, 172–4
Berry D, 211
Bewley C, 189–90
Bhavnani K-K, 16
Billington R, 130
Blaxter M, 50–1, 57
Blazer D, 61
Bloor M, 85
Bordo S, 181
Botting B, 49
Bourdieu P, 3, 44–7, 100
Bowden P, 113, 118–22, 217
Bowlby J, 31
Brannon R, 36, 60
Briggs A, 67–8, 95, 97
Brittain V, 84
Brockbank W, 73
Broom L, 7
Broverman I K, 9, 15
Brown G, 57, 191
Brown J, 152
Brown R G S, 103
Browne A, 209
Bruce E, 220–2
Bruch H, 180–1
Buchan J, 11
Bunting J, 187
Bunting S, 166
Burstow B, 171
Bury M, 194–5, 222
Busfield J, 9, 13–15, 25, 43–4,
    50, 53, 57–8, 61, 128, 181,
    209
Butler J, 26

C

Cameron E, 63, 172–4
Campbell J, 213
Campbell J C, 166
Canaan J E, 40–1
Canetto S, 187–8
Carpenter M, 28, 78, 80

Cavanagh J T O, 188
Chambers M, 107
Champagne J, 42
Charles J, 194
Charles N, 192–4, 197
Charmaz K, 195–7
Chesler P, 53
Chinn P L, 165
Chinoy E, 7
Chodorow N, 129
Cixous H, 101, 120
Clancy C M, 63
Clark D C, 188
Clark J Mcleod, 140
Clark P, 162
Collins P Hill, 16, 24, 33
Collinson D L, 148
Colyer H, 205–6
Connell R W, 14, 16, 26, 30,
    40, 115, 172
Cook E P, 9–10
Cornwall A, 172
Cowan P J, 182
Coyle J, 178, 206
Cribb A, 140
Curtis L, 194

D
Dahl T, 219
Dalley G, 123
Dally A, 81
Dalton K, 190
Daly M, 58
Davies C, 2, 9–10, 14–15, 18,
    28–30, 69, 105–6, 119, 130,
    136–9, 141, 148–50, 220
Davis M A, 52–3
Delphy C, 23
Department of Health, 112,
    122, 154–5, 157, 187, 193
Department of Social Security,
    56
Dines A, 140
Dingwall R, 70–1, 74, 76–7,
    84, 86–9
Dobash R E, 212
Dolan B, 107
Dominelli L, 166

Donald J, 116
Doyal L, 48, 50–1, 54, 58, 61,
    99, 170
Drever F, 187
Dunnell K, 49

E
Edwards A, 15
Egeland J, 152
Ehrenreich B, 217
Eisler R M, 60
Eisner M, 169–70
Eliasson R, 221
Ellerby K, 107
Engels F, 19
English D, 217
Epstein D, 36
Etzioni A, 8
Evandrou M, 56
Evans J, 106, 151–3

F
Farnworth M, 98
Farr K A, 186
Feeney A, 56
Ferguson K, 211
Few C, 203
Finch J, 122–3
Finkelhor D, 209
Firestone S, 21–2
Foster P, 206
Foucault M, 118
Fox N, 118, 120
Franks P, 63
Frazier F, 43
Freud S, 128, 185
Friedan B, 21

G
Gamarnikow E, 18, 28
General Nursing Council, 87,
    89–90
Geertz C, 130
Giddens A, 2
Gilbert N, 123, 220–1
Gilligan C, 28, 119–20, 222
Gilligan J, 214
Gilloran A, 154, 157

Gilmore D, 39
Godfrey J, 36
Goffman E, 19, 20
Goleman D, 126, 155
Gordon D F, 173, 204
Gordon M, 192
Gordon R A, 180
Gove W R, 54
Graham H, 57, 123, 218–20, 223
Gramsci A, 30
Grant G, 56
Green H, 221
Greene J, 88
Gregoire A J P, 190
Gregor F, 219
Greipp M E, 162–3
Grimwood C, 154
Groves D, 122

H
Hadley S, 213
Hagell E I, 165
Halford S, 102, 106, 148–9
Hallam J, 92–3, 96, 107–8
Hammersley M, 167
Hannam J, 79
Hargreaves J, 36
Harris T, 57, 191
Harrison M J, 223–5
Hearn J, 16, 148, 186, 214–16
Heinrich K T, 165
Helgeson V, 59–61
Henderson V, 111
Heulskoetter M, 183
Hochschild A, 124–6, 131–3
Holden J, 189, 193
Holland S, 171–2
Holley C, 211
Hollin C R, 183
Holloway W, 150
Holme A, 222
Holmes P, 107
Holt R, 38
hooks b, 170
Horrocks R, 62
House J S, 61
House of Commons, 87

Hughes D, 134
Humphreys J, 213
Hunt K, 59–60
Hunt S, 191
Hutt R, 105

I
Ireland J, 104, 106–7

J
James N, 28, 111, 124–5, 158, 220
Jezierski M, 213
Johnson M, 153
Jones K, 102–3
Jones L, 205
Jones M, 106
Julien I, 43
Juni S, 60

K
Kahan B, 212
Kalisch B J, 92
Kalisch P A, 92
Kant E, 34
Kanter R, 151–2
Kaufman-Kanter G, 190
Kauppinen-Toropainen K, 152
Kaye L W, 225
Keddy B C, 165
Kelleher D, 195
Kendall S, 140
Kendall-Thakett K A, 190
Kennell J H, 189
Kenny T, 180
Kerfoot D, 155–6
Kintz L, 38
Kirkham M, 168–9
Kitzinger J, 210
Kitzinger S D, 190
Klaus M H, 189
Klein M, 128
Klein V, 93–7
Knights K, 155–6
Komarovsky M, 97
Kondo D K, 130
Kuhse H, 28, 112, 120

L
Lammi J, 152
Lask S, 140
Latter S, 140
Lawler J, 26, 199–200
Lawrence M, 180
Lee R M, 126
Lee Treweek G, 125, 208
Lees S, 35
Levy A, 212
Lewis J, 122
Lindisfarne N, 172
Lister R, 39, 56, 121–2
Littlewood J, 189–90, 193–4
Lloyd W A, 104–5, 150–1, 157
Lodge N, 201–2
Long C G, 183
Lorber J, 51, 63
Luker K A, 205
Lukes S, 201
Lumby J, 206–8

M
Mac an Ghaill M, 16, 40
MacDougall G, 162, 175
Macintyre S, 33, 48, 52–3, 203, 220
Mackay L, 113–14, 134–5, 163
Maggs C, 70, 72–3, 76, 80
Mama A, 212
Marmot M, 56
Marsland L, 103–4
McGown A, 184
McHugh N, 189–90, 193–4
McKie L, 202
McIntosh J, 85, 193
McLeer S, 212
Mead G H, 20
Medico-Psychological Association, 89
Meltzer H, 50
Menzies I, 147
Mercer K, 43
Meredith B, 122
Messner M, 186
Middleton S, 98–101
Miers M, 54, 68, 86, 138, 164, 205

Miles A, 48, 206
Millett K, 128
Milligan F, 69, 88, 103–4
Mills C Wright, 217
Ministry of Health, Scottish Home and Health Department, 104, 146, 148–9
Minuchin S, 180
Moore J, 78
Morris J, 122–3, 170
Murray M, 107
Murray R, 183
Myrdal A, 93–7

N
National Asylum Workers Union, 89
Neufeld A, 223–5
Newton L H, 113
Nicolson P, 33, 191
Nightingale Florence, 37, 73, 82, 88
Noddings N, 217
Nolan M, 56
Nolan P, 103, 176
Nuttal P, 105

O
Oakley A, 1–2, 4, 9, 20, 32–3, 54, 167, 191
Oates M, 193
Office for National Statistics, 49–50, 204
Orbach S, 129, 139, 181
Oribabor P, 82–3
Ozga J, 154

P
Pahl J, 212–13, 215
Parker G, 123
Parkin W, 200–1
Parrish J, 96
Parsons T, 17–18, 194
Payne S, 218
Pearson A, 112, 141
Pennebaker J W, 61
Perry P, 156

Phillips D, 164
Phoenix A, 33
Phoenix P, 16
Piani A, 50
Piper S, 162, 174
Pleck J H, 60
Plumwood V, 15
Popplestone R, 154
Porter S, 8, 17, 21, 86, 102, 106, 134–6
Pringle R, 15, 150
Pringle M Kellmer, 12–13
Pronger B, 37
Purves L, 174

R
Ramazonoglu C, 167
Ratcliffe P, 153
Reverby S, 113
Rhodes P, 202
Richardson D, 16, 31–2
Roberts H, 206
Roberts S, 152, 182
Robinson I, 195
Robinson V, 16
Rodwell C, 140
Romans P, 33
Rose H, 221–2
Rosen J G, 102–3
Rosser J, 28, 105
Rousseau J, 120
Ruddick S, 217
Russell G F M, 180
Ryan S, 106

S
Sabo D, 173
Salvage J, 112
Savage J, 141
Savage M, 15
Schoenborn C, 50
Schroeder M A, 183
Segal L, 203
Seidler V, 34
Selznick P, 7
Shajahan P M, 188
Sharp K, 161
Sheehan A, 211

Simonen L, 221
Simson M, 98
Skeggs B, 9, 35, 37–8, 100–1, 115–18
Skidmore J R, 60
Sloan G, 183
Smart C, 36
Smith Pam, 28, 125, 163
Smith Paul, 42
Snare A, 219
Sofer C, 147
Spence J, 35
Spence J T, 59
Stacey J, 21
Stanley L, 167
Stanworth M, 58
Staples R, 43
Stein L, 8, 133–4, 136, 220
Stillion J M, 53, 187
Stones R W H, 103
Stryker S, 20
Sturt J, 141
Sullivan A, 175
Summers A, 72–6
Symonds A, 191

T
Tait A, 171
Taylor B M, 203
Taylor F W, 157, 203
Taylor H, 57, 203
Tewksbury R, 176–7
Tickle L, 49
Tiefer L, 202
Tilt E, 37
Tones K, 140
Trobst K, 61
Tudor J F, 54
Twomey M, 168

U
Ungerson C, 122–3
United Kingdom Central Council for Nursing, Midwifery and Health Visiting, 140, 217
Ussher J, 190

V
Valentine P, 153, 182
Vandeemer Y G, 190
Ve H, 220
Villeneuve M, 152

W
Walby S, 24, 136
Waldron I, 48, 50
Wallace C, 7–8, 22, 24, 162
Walters E, 184
Walters V, 35, 191–2, 197
Wardhaugh J, 201
Watson G, 171
Watson J, 112–13, 118
Webb C, 167–8, 205
Webb D, 126
Weber M, 146, 149
Weeks J, 42, 179
Wenger N K, 63
West P, 203
Wheeler C E, 165
Whitbread J, 184
White H, 187
White J, 183
White P G, 185–6
White R, 85, 98–100, 143–8
Whitehead L, 184
Whitley B E, 60
Whitton A, 193
Wilding P, 201

Wilkinson G, 86
Wilkinson R G, 214
Williams C, 103
Williams C L, 152, 175
Williams G, 195
Williams J, 171
Williams S J, 195
Willis P, 40
Wilson-Barnett J, 168
Wilton T, 177, 179
Winship J, 35
Witt B, 165
Wittgenstein L, 118
Wittig M, 23, 179
Witz A, 15, 28, 86–7, 137–8
Wollstonecraft M, 21
Woodward J, 71
Worsley P, 7
Wright M, 169–70
Wrubel J, 112–13, 118, 125, 198

Y
York University Students
  Union, 7, 11
Young E H, 126

Z
Zaretsky E, 19
Zola I, 219

Subject Index

A

abuse, 210–12
adolescence, 180–4
anorexia nervosa *see* eating
  disorders
arthritis, 195, 197–8
asylum attendants, 76, 80
asylums, 77, 89
authority, 146
autonomy, 137, 139

B

biological explanations for
  gender differences, 12
breast cancer, 170
Briggs Report of the
  Committee on Nursing,
  67–8, 95
bulimia *see* eating disorders
bureaucracy, 148–9

C

capitalism, 16, 23, 181
care/caring, 55, 100, 114–16,
  118–28, 131, 158, 161–77,
  182, 220
  and curriculum, 100
  and ethics, 119–21
  and social status, 128, 131
  care as discipline, 118, 120
  care as gift, 118, 120
  carework, 125, 158
  community care, 122, 219
  gender-sensitive care, 161–77
  informal care, 123, 220
  woman-centred care, 182, 211
  'vigil of care', 118
caring, 55, 114–16
  and health, 55
  and respectability, 115
  and responsibility, 114–15
  caring self, 114–16

childbirth *see* pregnancy
citizen/citizenship, 121–2
chronic illness, 172, 194–5
class, 80, 81, 97
  and curriculum, 100
  and health, 56
  and nursing *see* nursing and
    class
  measurements of, 56
cognitive behavioural therapy,
  183
community nursing, 168, 193
Crimean war, 72, 74, 80
cultural capital, 44–7
cultural codes, 10, 28–30, 35

D

dependency, 139
depression, 188–91
disability, 122–3
discourse, 25, 108
disempowerment, 178, 206,
  208
doctors/doctor–nurse
  relationship *see* medical
  profession
domestic labour/domestic work,
  18, 19, 24
dominance, 36
dual systems theory, 22, 24

E

eating disorders, 180–4
Edinburgh Postnatal Depression
  Scale, 138
education, 86, 93, 98, 100,
  115–16, 145, 156, 165
  caring courses, 100, 115–16
  nurse education, 86, 138,
    145, 165
  for women, 93, 98, 156
emotional intelligence, 126, 155

emotional labour, 111, 124–6, 131–3
empathy, 60–1
empowerment, 141–2
ethics, 119–21

F
family therapy, 182
father, 34–5
feeling rules, 126
feminine/femininities, 10, 35, 54, 61, 79, 81, 93–4, 98–100
feminisms, 20–4, 57, 79, 164–6, 216
feminist research, 166
food, 181, 218–19
functionalism, 17–18, 161–2

G
gender, 9–16, 26–7, 48, 53, 57, 125–7, 148, 212–14
  and the body, 15
  and care, 125–7
  and health, 48, 53, 57
  and organisations, 148
  and power, 16, 212–14
  and sexuality, 16, 212–14
  as a binary category, 13
  as a cultural/social construction, 13, 26–30, 35, 68, 127
  as a linking concept, 14
  bias in care delivery, 162–3
  key features, 9, 13, 29
gender differences, 10
gender dsyphoria, 184
gender identity, 15–16, 179, 184–5
gender inequalities, 14
gender order, 26, 30, 48, 175
gender-sensitive care, 121, 161–216
general practitioners *see* medical profession

H
handy-women, 69–70

health, 54–6, 172–4, 203
  and employment/ unemployment, 54, 56
  and femininity, 54
  and masculinity, 60–1, 172–4, 204
  sexual health, 203
Health and Lifestyle Survey, 57
health promotion, 140
health visitors/visiting, 85, 213
heart disease, 51
hegemony, 30
hegemonic masculinity, 30–1
heterosexuality, 36, 179, 203
hierarchy/hierarchical, 78, 81, 83, 215
HIV/AIDS, 175–6
homosexuality, 38, 176–7
hospital management committees, 144
hospitals, 71, 144, 147
housewife/housework, 20, 33, 54, 94

I
identity(ies), 114, 178
  and chronic illness, 178, 194
  sex-role identity, 15
ideological projects, 31, 46–7, 79
  capitalist, 42, 44
  heterosexual, 42
  knowledge, 44, 79, 91, 118, 136
  management, 43
  morality, 42, 46
  patriarchal, 42
illness experience, 194–8, 204, 208
imperialism, 43
instrumental/instrumentality, 10
interactionism/interactionist, 19–20, 216

J
justice, 119–21

L
Local Government Act 1986, 42

M
'malestream' sociology, 7, 18
management, 143–50
    men in nursing management, 104, 150–5
management style, 153–5
manliness, 38
Marxism, 19
masculinity(ies), 10, 30, 36, 40, 61, 81, 107, 152, 173
    and health, 60–1, 172–4, 204
    hegemonic masculinity, 30–1, 172
    marginalised masculinity, 172, 176
    negative, 60
    positive, 59–60
    trait masculinity, 59
matron, 82–3, 143–7
medical profession, 77, 87, 102, 106, 133–6
    doctor–nurse relationships, 77–8, 102, 106, 133–6
    general practitioners, 169–70, 203
    medical superintendents, 76, 89
medicalisation/demedicalisation, 82–3, 183, 193
men in nursing 13, 75, 87–90, 102, 106, 153–4, 175
Mental Deficiency Act 1913, 89
mental illness/ health, 55–8, 171
mental nurses *see* psychiatric nursing
midwifery, 168–9, 201
morality project *see* ideological projects
morbidity, 50–3
mortality rates, 48–50
mother/motherhood, 31–3, 38, 96, 130, 189–92

N
Nightingale fund, 75
Nurse Registration Bill, 87, 137
nursing/nurses, 11, 16, 69–90, 92–3, 95–8, 101–3, 105, 111, 138, 140, 143–58, 175
    and armed services, 74, 102
    and class, 69–70, 72–80, 87, 93
    and romance, 70, 92, 101
    and sexuality, 11, 16, 92, 101
    and sisters in charge, 72
    and spiritual care, 72
    development as a profession, 85–90
    education and training, 86, 98, 138
    history, 69–90
    management, 105, 143–58
    in the media, 68, 92
    primary, 140
    private, 69–70
    process, 111
    pupil (enrolled status), 97
    recruitment, 68–72, 95–7, 103
    sisterhoods, 71–2, 83
    stereotypes, 11, 68, 92
    student (registered status), 97

O
object relations theory, 128
Oedipus complex, 185
older people, 221–5
oppression/oppressed group, 23, 152, 177, 179
organisation, 148–50, 155
organising, 2, 158
other-orientation, 131

P
particularism, 17
patriarchy, 16, 23–4, 42, 164, 203
police, 214–15
poor law hospitals, 82
post-Fordism, 155

postmodernism, 25, 47
postnatal depression, 189–94
power/powerlessness, 23, 152,
    177–9, 201, 206–9
pregnancy and childbirth, 189,
    192–3, 210
profession/professionalism, 136
    new professionalism, 130,
    138–9
professionalising project, 137–8
Project 2000, 138
prostate disease, 173
Prostate Help Association, 173
public school, 38
psychiatric nursing, 97, 103–4,
    176, 193, 209
psychotherapy, 172

Q
queer theory, 25–6

R
rational/rationality, 39, 44
reciprocity, 221–3
registration campaign, 86–7
respectability/responsibility, 35,
    39, 70, 78–9, 83, 114

S
Salmon Report of the
    Committee on Senior Nursing
    Structure, 104, 146, 148–9
self/self-concept, 3
    caring self, 114–16
self-efficacy, 141

self-esteem, 183
self-orientation, 139
sex-role, 15
sexual harassment, 199
sexuality, 25–6, 99, 119–200,
    204
shell-shock, 209
'sisterhoods' see nursing
smoking, 57
social role, 17, 14
social support, 61
sport, 185–6
    and masculinity, 38–9
subordination, 131, 140
suicide and suicidal acts, 187–9
surveillance, 85

T
testicular cancer, 205
transexualism, 184

V
Victorian culture, 113, 147
    constructions of femininity,
    79, 81, 113
violence, 61, 212–14
Voluntary Aid Detachments
    (VADs), 84

W
woman-centred care/therapy,
    182, 211
women's changing role, 95–8
    'good woman', 37, 117, 211